PANDEMIC HISTORY

The Worst Pandemics That
Changed History

John Muan

Copyright @ 2020 by John Muan - All rights reserved.

This book is written with the sole purpose of providing relevant information on a specific topic for which every reasonable effort has been made to ensure that it is both accurate and reasonable. Nevertheless, by purchasing this book you consent to the fact that the author, as well as the publisher, are in no way experts on the topics contained herein, regardless of any claims as such that may be made within. As such, any suggestions or recommendations that are made within are done so purely for entertainment value. It is recommended that you always consult a professional, prior to undertaking any of the advice or techniques discussed within.

This is a legally binding declaration that is considered both valid and fair by both the Committee of Publishers Association and the American Bar Association and should be considered as legally binding within the United States.

The reproduction, transmission, and duplication of any of the content found herein, including any specific or extended information will be done as an illegal act regardless of the end form the information ultimately takes. This includes copied versions of the work both physical, digital and audio unless express consent of the Publisher is provided beforehand. Any additional rights reserved.

Furthermore, the information that can be found within the pages described forthwith shall be considered both accurate and truthful when it comes to the recounting of facts. As such, any use, correct or incorrect, of the provided information will render the Publisher free of responsibility as to the actions taken outside of their direct purview. Regardless, there are zero scenarios where the original author or the Publisher can be deemed liable in any fashion for any damages or hardships that may result from any of the information discussed herein.

Additionally, the information in the following pages is intended only for informational purposes and should thus be thought of as universal. As befitting its nature, it is presented without assurance regarding its prolonged validity or interim quality. Trademarks that are mentioned are done without written consent and can in no way be considered an endorsement from the trademark holder.

TABLE OF CONTENTS

INTRODUCTION 7
CHAPTER 1 - MALARIA 9
   Brief History of Malaria 9
   The Existing Pattern of the Malaria Parasites, Plasmodium Spp 14
   The Malaria Parasites 16
   Transmission 21
CHAPTER 2 – TUBERCULOSIS 25
   History of Tuberculosis 25
   Transmission 29
      Do vampires cause TB? 29
   Finding TB Is the Initial Move Towards Ending TB 30
   Vaccine 32
   Treatment 32
CHAPTER 3 - HISTORY OF SMALLPOX 35
   Origin of Smallpox 35
   Spread of Smallpox 35
   Early Control Efforts 36
   Worldwide Smallpox Eradication Program 38
   Last Cases of Smallpox 39
   World Free of Smallpox 41
   Stocks of Variola Virus 42
CHAPTER 4 - PLAGUE AND BLACK DEATH (1346-1353) 43
CHAPTER 5 - CHOLERA 53
   Illness & Symptoms 53
   Sources of Infection and Risk Factors 55
   Diagnosis and Detection 55

The Most Effective Method to Diagnose 56
Suspected Cholera Case 57
Confirmed Cholera Case 57
Quick Tests 57
Treatment 58
    Cholera Treatments 58
CHAPTER 6 - SPANISH INFLUENZA (1918-20) 61
    History of 1918 Flu Pandemic (Española) 62
    The Global Death Count of the Flu Today 64
    Worldwide Deaths of the Spanish Flu 65
    Other Large Influenza Pandemics 67
    The Effect of the Spanish Influenza Pandemic on Various Age Groups 68
    Plague Origination and Transmission 72
    Kinds of Plague and Symptoms 74
CHAPTER 7 - THE SPREAD OF THE PLAGUE THROUGH THE BYZANTINE EMPIRE 77
    Plague Treatment 79
    Impacts on the Byzantine Empire 80
CHAPTER 8 - HONG KONG FLU (1968 INFLUENZA PANDEMIC) 82
    Hong Kong Flu History 82
    A World Health Organization Report 86
CHAPTER 9 - HIV AND AIDS 89
    Successes in HIV Prevention 93
    Remaining Challenges 95
    New Strategies 97
    Special Issue of MMWR 102
    The Development of Research, Treatment, and Prevention 103
    Current Treatment 104

The Social Reaction to HIV 105
   Stigma in the Early Years 105
Government Support.. 106
Mainstream Society Opens Up Discussions About HIV 106
Following the Legislative Issues of Blood Bans 107
Ongoing Medication Advancement for HIV Prevention............... 108
What Impact Does HIV Have on the Body?................................... 109
How Is HIV Transmitted?... 110
What Are the Phases of HIV?.. 111
   HIV Is Characterized by 3 Phases: Acute HIV, Chronic HIV, and AIDS... 111
   How Does Chronic HIV Influence the Body?................................. 113

CHAPTER 10 - SERIOUS ACUTE RESPIRATORY SYNDROME (SARS)... 115

The Making of a Crisis... 118
What Is the Cause of SARS?...122
What Are SARS Risk Factors?..123
What Are the Signs and Symptoms of SARS?................................123
When Should Someone Seek Medical Care for Possible Exposure to SARS? 124
What Specialists Treat SARS?..125
What Tests Do Physicians Use to Diagnose SARS? 125
Are There Home Remedies for SARS?..126
What Are SARS Treatments? 127
What Medications Treat SARS?...127
How Often Is Follow-up Needed After SARS Treatment?.............128
By What Means Can People Prevent SARS? 128
What Is the Prognosis for SARS?...130
The 2009 H1N1 Pandemic: A New Flu Virus Emerges.................. 131

CHAPTER 11 - EBOLA 135
What Are the Side Effects of Ebola? 135
Is Ebola Treatable? 135
How Is Ebola Spread? 136
For What Reason Did the 2014 Outbreak in West Africa Spread So Quickly? 137
For What Reason Was Ebola So Difficult to Stop? 137
Is There a Risk of an Ebola Episode in the United States? 138
How might I help survivors of Ebola? 139
World Vision's Reaction to the Ebola Outbreak 139
Health and Safety 140
Awareness and Prevention 140
Safe and Dignified Burials 141
Social and Economic Recovery 142

CHAPTER 12 - PANDEMIC RISK FACTORS 145
Spark Risk 145
Spread Risk 146
Burden of Pandemics 148
Consequences of Pandemics 150
Health Impacts 150
Economic Impacts 154
Social and Political Impacts 156
Patterns Affecting Pandemic Risk 158

CONCLUSION 161

INTRODUCTION

Epidemics, plagues, and pandemics have been around since the beginning of progress. Without a doubt, they are an unintended result of civilization. Infection certainly afflicted our prehistoric ancestors, however, since the earliest people lived in little isolated groups, they had restricted chance to share germs beyond their locality. That circumstance changed drastically when the agricultural revolution replaced roaming with a sedentary way of life 10,000 years prior. Sickness and diseases have plagued humanity since the most punctual days of our mortal flaw. But, it was not until the marked move to agrarian communities that the scale and spread of these infections increased dramatically. Across the board, the exchange made new chances for human and creature connections that sped up to such epidemics. Malaria, tuberculosis, leprosy, influenza, smallpox, and others initially showed up during these early years. The more enlightened people became, with bigger urban communities, more exotic trade courses, and expanded contact with various populations of individuals, animals, and environments, the almost certain pandemics would happen. Despite the persistence of disease and pandemics since the beginning, there's one steady pattern after some time, which is a continuous decrease in the death rate. Healthcare improvements and understanding the variables that hatch pandemics have been incredible assets in relieving their effect. Despite his apparent knowledge of the role geography and exchange played in this spread, Procopius laid the fault for the outbreak on the Emperor Justinian, announcing him to be either a devil or invoking God's punishment for his evil ways. A few history specialists found that this occasion could have run Emperor Justinian's efforts to rejoin the Western and Eastern remainders of the Roman Empire and denoted the start of the Dark Ages.

CHAPTER 1 - MALARIA

Brief History of Malaria

Malaria involves one of a kind spot in the records of history. Over centuries, its victims have included Neolithic occupants, early Chinese and Greeks, poor people, and royalty. Just in the twentieth century, malaria asserted between 150 million and 300 million lives, representing 2 to 5 percent of all deaths. Although its main sufferers today are the poor of sub-Saharan Africa, Asia, the Amazon basin, and other tropical districts, 40 percent of the total population despite everything lives in areas where malaria is transmitted.

Ancient works and artifacts vouch for malaria's long rule. Dirt tablets with cuneiform content from Mesopotamia notice deadly periodic fevers suggestive of malaria. Malaria antigen was, as of late, identified in the Egyptian remains dating from 3200 and 1304 BC. Indian works of the Vedic time frame (1500 to 800 BC) considered malaria the "king of diseases." In 270 BC, the Chinese clinical group known as the Nei Chin connected tertian (each third day) and quartan (each fourth day) fevers with the extension of the spleen (a typical finding in jungle fever), and accused malaria's headaches, chills, and fevers on three evil demons; one carrying a hammer, another a bucket of water, and the third a stove.

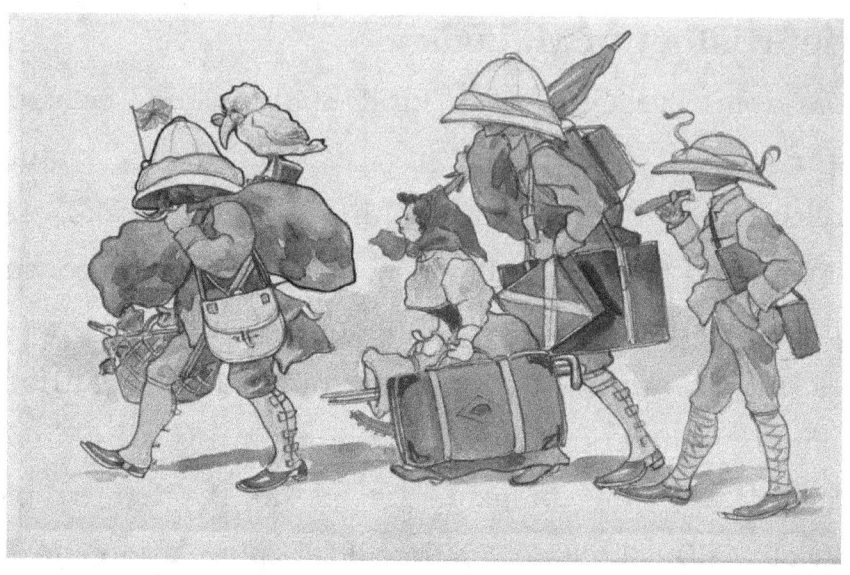

1 Terzi, A. J, E. 1872-1956[1]

The Greek artist Homer (around 750 BC) refers to malaria in The Iliad, as does Aristophanes (445-385 BC) in The Wasps, and Aristotle (384-322 BC), Plato (428-347 BC), and Sophocles (496-406 BC). Like Homer, Hippocrates (450-370 BC) connected the presence of Sirius, the canine star (in pre-fall and pre-winter) with malarial fever and misery.

Malaria's likely appearance in Rome in the primary century AD was a defining moment in European history.

---

[1] Three members of the Roman Campagne Malaria Commission with a lady carrying their gear. Coloured pen drawing by A. Terzi, ca 1900 -
https://wellcomecollection.org/works/w5rczz8g

From the African rain forest, the disease no doubt traveled down the Nile to the Mediterranean, and then, spread east to the Fertile Crescent and north to Greece. Greek colonists and traders carried it to Italy. From that point, Roman officers and merchants would look like at last carry it as far north as England and Denmark.

For the following 2,000 years, any place Europe harbored swarmed settlements and standing water, malaria flourished, rendering people regularly sick, and incessantly powerless and detached. Numerous history students theorize that *falciparum malaria* (the deadliest type of jungle fever species in people) added to the fall of Rome. The malaria epidemic of 79 AD crushed the prolific, marshy croplands surrounding the city, making local farmers surrender their fields and towns. As late as the nineteenth century, explorers to these equivalent areas commented on the weakness of the population, their sordid life, and miserable agriculture. The Roman Campagna would remain inadequately settled until at last freed from malaria in the late 1930s.

In India and China, populace development drove individuals into semitropical southern areas that supported malaria. India's most seasoned settled locale was the relatively dry Indus valley to the north. Migrants to the hot, wet Ganges valley toward the south were disproportionately plagued by malaria and other mosquito-and water-borne illnesses. A huge number of workers who left the Yellow River for hot and sticky rice paddies bordering the Yangtze experienced comparative dangers. Because of the inconsistent burden of disease, for centuries, the advancement of China's south was behind its north.

Although a few researchers guess that *vivax malaria* may have gone with the most punctual New World immigrants who showed up using the Bering Strait, there are no records of malaria in the Americas before European adventurers, conquistadores, and settlers carried *Plasmodium malaria*, and *P. vivax* as microscopic cargo. *Falciparum malaria* was, in this way, imported to the New World by African slaves at first secured by age-old genetic defenses (sickle cell iron deficiency and G6PD insufficiency), and in addition to partial immunity gained through the deep-rooted presentation. Their relatives, just as Native Americans and pioneers of European lineage, were more defenseless, however. Deforestation and "wet" horticulture, for example, rice cultivating, encouraged the reproduction of *Anopheles* mosquitoes. By 1750, both vivax and falciparum malaria were basic from the tropics of Latin America to the Mississippi valley to New England.

Malaria, both epidemic and endemic, kept on plague the United States until the mid-twentieth century. It struck presidents from Washington to Lincoln, and debilitated several thousand Civil War fighters (in 1862, Washington, D.C.). Its environmental factors were malarious to the point that General McClellan's Army in transit to Yorktown was stopped in its tracks, traveled to California with the Gold Rush. He guaranteed Native American lives over the continent. Until the Tennessee Valley Authority carried hydroelectric force and modernization to the country South during the 1930s, malaria depleted the physical and financial well-being of the whole district. Similarly, as the United States was destroying its last indigenous pockets of disease, intestinal sickness became Americans' consideration during World War II. During the beginning of the Pacific campaign, more soldiers tumbled to malaria than to enemy forces. The United States' chief general well-being office—the Centers for Disease Control and Prevention—was established in light of malaria.

During the Vietnam War, the American military found that the drug-resistant malaria was at that point across the board in Southeast Asia, a harbinger of the global danger it was bound to turn into.

However, no place, past or present, has malaria demanded a more prominent cost than in Africa. A groundbreaking guarded pathogen was the main obstacle to Africa's colonization. Portuguese traders who entered the African seaside plain in the late 1400s and mid-1500s were the principal outsiders to stand up to the killing fever. For the following 3 centuries, at whatever point European forces tried to build up stations on the continent, they were repelled consistently by malaria, yellow fever, and other tropical scourges. By the eighteenth century, the dark specter of disease earned West and focal Africa the famous inscription, "the White Man's Grave."

The Existing Pattern of the Malaria Parasites, Plasmodium Spp

To understand the historical events, it is important to summarize our present condition of information quickly. Malaria is brought about by contamination with five types of *Plasmodium*, the existing patterns of which are fundamentally the same.

Contamination starts when *sporozoites*, the infective stages, are infused by a mosquito and are carried around the body until they attack liver *hepatocytes*, where they experience a phase of asexual multiplication (*exoerythrocytic schizogony*), bringing about the creation of numerous uninucleate *merozoites*. These *merozoites* flood out into the blood and attack red blood cells, where they start the second period of a phase of asexual multiplication (*erythrocytic schizogony*), bringing about the creation of around 8-16 *merozoites* which attack new red blood cells. This procedure is repeated uncertainly and is liable for the disease, malaria. As the infection advances, some youthful *merozoites* form into male and female *gametocytes* that flow in the peripheral blood until they are taken up by a female *anopheline mosquito* when it bites a victim. Inside the mosquito, the *gametocytes* develop into male and female gametes, fertilization happens, and a *motile zygote* (*ookinete*) is formed inside the lumen of the mosquito gut, signaling the start of a procedure known as *sporogony*. The *ookinete* penetrates the gut wall and turns into a prominent *oocyst* inside which another period of increase happens to bring about the arrangement of *sporozoites* that relocate to the salivary organs of a mosquito and are infused when the mosquito bites another host.

The Malaria Parasites

Our understanding of the malaria parasites' life cycle didn't continue in the legitimate request simply delineated; however, more like a jigsaw, The different pieces were meticulously instituted and similar to a jigsaw, that frequently involved mistakes and false starts. The story starts with the disclosure of the phases in the blood. Numerous course readings only express that 'in 1880 Laveran found the malaria parasite' words that don't give this revelation the credit it deserves. To understand the foundation of this revelation, it is important to return to the 1870s. The revelations of Pasteur and Koch had accelerated a search for a bacterial reason for many diseases, including malaria. By 1879 the miasma hypothesis was leaving favor, and the two theories competing for conflict were whether the microorganisms responsible were transmitted via air and inhalation or by water and ingestion. The main hypothesis was that proposed by the Italian Corrado Tommasi-Crudeli and the German Theodor Albrecht Edwin Klebs, a prominent microbiologist who had been the primary person to see the microscopic organisms answerable for typhoid and diphtheria.

Tommasi-Crudeli and Klebs guaranteed that they had isolated from the waters of the Pontine Marshes, where jungle fever was predominant, the bacterium, *Bacillus malariae*, which when segregated in culture and infused into rabbits caused febrile diseases joined by developed spleens reminiscent of malaria. It was against this foundation that Charles Louis Alphonse Laveran, an unknown French armed force official working in Algeria, tested the apparent insight and started in his own words 'to follow the pigment.' Starting with the well-established actuality that the spleens of intestinal sickness patients contained shade, he started to search for color in the fresh unstained blood of patients and watched it first in quite a while and then in or on red blood cells. Looking all the more cautiously, he watched a few unique types of *erythrocytic* life forms, including sickles, round motionless bodies with pigment, circular moving bodies with shade, and bodies that expelled flagella-like structures, all of which he thought were outward of outside of the red cells.

These perceptions are especially interesting because Laveran utilized fresh blood as well as a dry target with the greatest magnification of ×400 measurements. He also proposed a course of occasions that started with clear spots that developed, obtained color and filled the corpuscle, which at that point burst to match with the fevers related to malaria. Laveran carefully examined the blood of 200 patients and, in 148, watched the crescentic bodies in all instances of malaria yet never in those without jungle fever. He also noticed that quinine expelled these phases from the blood. Laveran quickly understood that he had discovered a parasitic protozoan, which he called *Oscillaria malariae*.

He introduced his discoveries to the French Academy of Medical Sciences in December 1880 but was unable to convince any of the prominent microbiologists, zoologists, or malariologists of the day that he saw something besides breaking down red cells. By and by, he drove forward and by 1884 had persuaded the main Italian malariologists, including Bignami, Golgi, and Marchiafava, that intestinal sickness was brought about by a protozoan and not a bacterium. His greatest success came around the same time when he also convinced the more critical microbiologists, Louis Pasteur, Charles Edouard Chamberland, and Pierre Paul Émile Roux. Robert Koch, one of the most influential microbiologists of his time, however, remained doubtful until 1887. By and by, in certain quarters, the miasma hypothesis endured. As late as 1895, the American R. C. Newton, a supporter of Tommasi-Crudeli, composed that 'Ethereal and oceanic transportation of malaria has been demonstrated.'

Laveran was granted the Nobel Prize for Medicine in 1907, and his revelations are depicted in some detail by the Sergent brothers and Bruce-Chwatt, just as in the different chronicles of malaria listed above.

What was surprising about Laveran's revelation was that it was unprecedented, as no protozoan had recently been found possessing any kind of human blood cell. Unbeknown to Laveran or the Italian malariologists, in any case, the Russian physiologist, Vassily Danilewsky had been looking at the blood of winged animals and reptiles in Ukraine and had found various parasites including *trypanosomes* and others that he recognized as '*pseudovacuoles.*' Any individual who has considered blood parasites will quickly perceive his description of '*pseudovacuoles*' as perfect malaria parasites. By 1885, Danilewsky had perceived the three most basic genera of *intraerythrocytic* blood parasites of feathered animals currently known as *Plasmodium, Haemoproteus*, and *Leucocytozoon*. However, as he had distributed a lot of his work in Russian, it was not until his three-volume book La Parasitologie Comparée du Sang had been distributed in French in 1889 that this data turned out to be generally available. From that point, there started scans for other malaria parasites in reptiles, winged animals, and warm-blooded animals, and this was encouraged by the accidental discovery of a methylene blue-eosin recolor by Dimitri Leonidovitch Romanowsky in 1891.

Romanowsky's stains got well known toward the start of the twentieth century and remain the premise of blood stains, for example, Leishman's, Giemsa's, and Wright's to the current day. These stains color the core of the nucleus red and the cytoplasm blue allowing their simple identifying proof and are utilized for jungle fever parasites as well as for *trypanosomes, leishmanias,* and filarial worms. Romanowsky's disclosure is one of the most critical specialized advances in the historical backdrop of parasitology.

Then the Italian specialists, presently convinced that malaria was caused by a parasite, responded to the call with power and Marchiafava and Bignami, utilizing a blend of eosin-based blood stains and the oil-immersion microscope objective created by the Carl Zeiss Company in 1882-4, watched *amoeboid* development of the living being. This left them in almost certainty that they were managing a protozoan parasite that attacked red cells, developed inside the cells, and delivered daughter cells that invaded fresh blood cells. From there on, the Italian perspectives dominated malaria research and, in the light of perceptions of the erythrocytic phases of the parasite,

Golgi between 1885-6 separated between tertian (48-hour periodicity) and quartan (72-hour periodicity) malaria and in 1889-1890, Golgi and Marchiafava further depicted the contrasts between mild Spring malaria (generous tertian) and extreme Summer-Autumn (dangerous tertian) malaria.

Transmission

Despite all their accumulated knowledge and skills, no malariologists could clarify how the parasite spread, starting with one human then onto the next. The clues were, moreover, set up. Throughout the hundreds of years, circumstantial evidence had amassed that recommended that mosquitoes may, in some way or another, be associated with malaria. By 1883, the American doctor, Albert King, had collected the mass of proof that was to get known as the mosquito-malaria doctrine. Somewhere in the range of 1884 and 1897, Laveran, Manson (who in 1877 had shown that the filarial worms responsible for *lymphatic filariasis* were transmitted by mosquitoes), and the Italian malariologists had become progressively convinced that mosquitoes were associated with the transmission of malaria. From that point, feelings compared with certain onlookers, including

Manson, accepting that people got tainted by drinking water contaminated by infected mosquitoes. In contrast, others felt that the disease was gained by breathing in dust from evaporated lakes in which contaminated mosquitoes died, and at the end of the day, a minor departure from the water and ingestion and air and inward breath hypotheses proposed by Tommasi-Crudeli and Klebs in 1879. Manson additionally played with the possibility that transmission may be mechanical; for example, the parasites were latently carried from host to be on the proboscis of a mosquito.

By 1894 Manson, who had spent quite a bit of his working life in Taiwan and was then in his 50s and had a built-up clinical practice in London, directed his attention toward the chance of mosquito transmission of malaria but, as he couldn't go to malarious countries himself, he required somebody to complete the fundamental examinations and investigations for him. His partner-to-be was an improbable decision, Ronald Ross

Ronald Ross, 1857-1932. In 1897 Ronald Ross was working in India and found that *culicine mosquitoes* transmitted the avian malaria parasite *Plasmodium relictum* and proposed that human malaria parasites may also be transmitted by mosquitoes. Afterward, when working in Sierra Leone in 1899, he published that the human malaria parasites were for sure transmitted by *anopheline mosquitoes*. Meanwhile, however, a few Italian researchers had just indicated this was the situation.

Ross, then aged 37, was a built-up army surgeon working in India who didn't accept that jungle fever was brought about by a blood parasite but believed that it was intestinal contamination. During the time half of 1894, Manson chipped away at Ross, gave him blood slides containing malaria parasites, and persuaded him that implicating a mosquito vector of malaria was an objective worth focusing on. Ross came back to India, and throughout the following four years, Manson coordinated tasks a good way off. We are lucky to have a practically complete variety of letters that went between the two men. This was not a simple relationship mostly because Ross's first needs were his military duties, and these definitely postponed the work he was doing with malaria and somewhat because, now and then, Ross appeared to be more interested in writing poetry and novels. By and by, the participation arrived at a good resolution; however, it later ended in acrimony.

CHAPTER 2 – TUBERCULOSIS

History of Tuberculosis

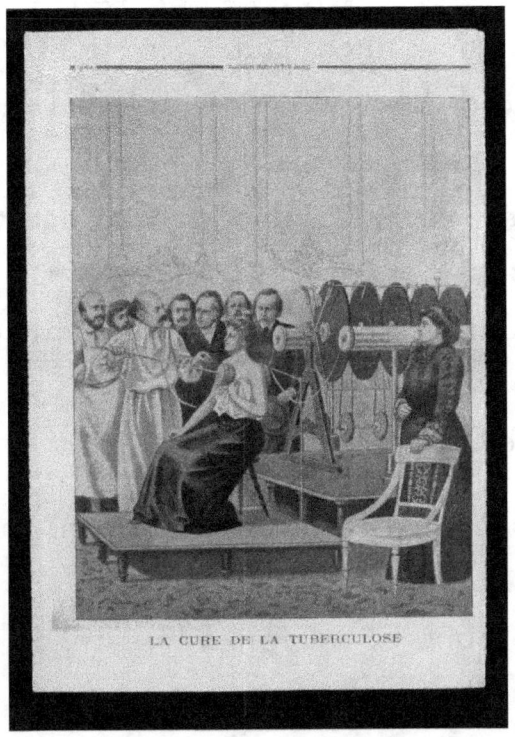

2 - La cure de la tuberculose[2]

TB in people can be followed back to 9,000 years prior in Atlit Yam, a city now under the Mediterranean Sea, off the bank of Israel. Archeologists discovered it in the remaining parts of a mother and child buried together.

---

[2] Francisque Crôtte applying his electrical remedy for tuberculosis to a seated woman. Colour process print, 1901
https://wellcomecollection.org/works/msvrfd75

The earliest written notices of TB were in India (3,300 years prior) and China (2,300 years back).

All through the 1600-1800s in Europe, TB caused 25% of death, everything being equal. Comparable numbers happened in the United States. In 1889, Dr. Hermann Biggs convinced the New York City Department of Health and Hygiene that specialists should report TB cases to the well-being office, prompting the main distributed report on TB in New York City in 1893. CDC distributed across the country TB information without precedent for 1953, revealing 84,304 instances of this infectious disease in the United States.

In 1867, tuberculosis (TB) was the main source of death in Canada. The bacterium that causes it, the tubercle *bacillus*, was found by a German researcher, Robert Koch, in 1882.

Verification that TB was contagious led to organized efforts to separate those tainted in sanatoria—unique clinics where patients could rest and get fresh air and a good diet.

The "rest cure" was the most widely recognized treatment for TB until anti-toxin treatment was created during the 1950s.

Another type of treatment was "collapse therapy." Surgeons pumped air into the chest pit so the lung could unwind, and the tuberculosis lesion could heal. The utilization of collapse treatment was first recorded in Ingersoll, Ontario, in 1898, yet it didn't become standard Canadian practice until 1919.

The main tuberculosis overview in Canada was led in 1921 by the Saskatchewan Anti-Tuberculosis Commission to decide the pace of disease among younger students. The study found that the greater part of the youngsters was infected with TB.

Mobile TB centers started in Ontario in 1923 and were before long utilized in each area. The clinics could diagnose, treat, and catch up with TB patients and their contacts. Portable x-beam machines could discover it before individuals indicated outer side effects, which made treatment far more effective.

Streptomycin was found in 1946—the main explicit anti-toxin that could slaughter the TB—causing bacterium. This and different anti-toxins turned out to be broadly utilized against TB during the 1950s.

Anti-infection treatment and a slight decrease in the occurrence of tuberculosis prompted shorter remains in sanatoria. The quantity of TB beds in Canada dropped from 18,977 in early 1953 to 9,722 out of 1963, and by the 1970s, just a few TB patients were admitted to the clinic.

Today, medical treatment is the main kind of treatment prescribed by doctors. However, guaranteeing that patients take the full course of medications, which, as a rule, requires a while, remains an issue.

TB is still thought to be one of the deadliest infectious diseases, especially in developing countries.

CDC distributes TB surveillance information on a yearly premise. In 2016, the latest information available, there were 9,272 reported cases of TB sickness in the United States. This sickness is a nationally notifiable disease; however, tuberculosis disease isn't reported to the CDC. CDC is exploring approaches to screen latent TB disease on a national premise. CDC has an objective of TB disposal in the United States. To arrive at this objective, CDC and partners are increasing the efforts to treat dormant tuberculosis infection in addition to TB disease.

Transmission

Do vampires cause TB?

Before the disclosure of the microscopic organisms that cause TB, the disease was believed to be genetic.

In the mid-1800s, there were "vampire panics" all through New England. At the point when a TB episode happened in a town, it was presumed that the principal relative to pass on of TB returned as a vampire to contaminate the remainder of the family. To stop the vampires, the townspeople would uncover the presumed vampire grave and play out a custom.

On March 24, 1882, Robert Koch declared his disclosure that TB was brought about by microorganisms in his introduction "Kick the bucket Aetiologie der Tuberculose" at the Berlin Physiological Society gathering. The disclosure of the microscopic organisms demonstrated that TB was an infectious disease, not hereditary. In 1905, Koch won the Nobel Prize for Medicine and Physiology.

Today, we realize TB is an airborne infectious disease, spread when an individual with TB illness hacks, talks, or sings. At the point when an individual is determined to have the disease, a contact examination is done to discover and test individuals (like relatives) who may have been presented to TB. Individuals determined to have TB ailment or inert TB Infection are then treated.

New technologies like entire genome sequencing help general well-being experts to see examples of TB transmission. This tool can help centralize general well-being efforts to discover and treat people with TB disease and idle TB disease.

Finding TB Is the Initial Move Towards Ending TB

The TB skin test for TB infection measures an individual's resistant reaction. The test is performed by infusing a limited quantity of liquid (called tuberculin) into the skin on the lower portion of the arm. A health care worker "reads" test after 72 hours.

The TB skin test was created after some time. In 1890, Robert Koch created tuberculin (an extract of the TB bacilli) as a fix; however, it ends up being inadequate. In 1907, Clemens von Pirquet built up a skin test that put a modest quantity of tuberculin under the skin and estimated the body's response. Pirquet additionally imagined the expression "idle TB contamination" in 1909.

In 1908, Charles Mantoux updated the skin test strategy by utilizing a needle and syringe to inject the tuberculin.

During the 1930s, American Florence Seibert Ph.D. built up a procedure to make a sanitized protein subordinate of tuberculin (PPD) for the TB skin test. Preceding this, the tuberculin utilized in skin tests was not steady or standardized. Seibert didn't patent the innovation, yet the United States government embraced it in 1940.

The TB skin test is still utilized today and has remained unaltered for very nearly eighty years. The test and PPD are still recorded on the World Health Organization's fundamental drugs list. A later progression in TB testing has been TB blood tests or interferon-gamma release assays (IGRAs).

Today, we utilize both TB skin tests and TB blood tests to analyze TB infection. Extra tests, similar to x-beams, are expected to analyze TB disease. At the point when TB was progressively endemic in the United States, public health departments frequently utilized versatile x-beam vans to test for TB. Mobile facilities are still being used today.

Testing and treating those in danger for TB is a key capacity of TB control programs in the United States and around the world.

Vaccine

Albert Calmette and Jean-Marie Camille Guerin built up the Bacille Calmette-Guérin (BCG) antibody in 1921. Before developing up the BCG vaccine, Calmette built up the first counter-agent to treat snake venom.

The BCG immunization isn't generally utilized in the United States, yet it is frequently given to babies and little kids to prevent TB meningitis in nations where TB is normal. BCG doesn't generally protect individuals from getting TB.

Vaccine investigation proceeds into what's to come. At the point when a more effective TB vaccine is created and conveyed, it could reduce infection and death the world over.

Treatment

Treatment remained largely unchanged until around 80 years back

Until the revelation of anti-toxins, treatment for TB was constrained to warmth, rest, and great nourishment... or "Lana, letto, latte" in Italian.

In the middle Ages, treatment for scrofula (TB of the lymph hubs and neck) was the "regal touch." People arranged for the royal touch of English and French rulers and queens, trusting a touch from the sovereign would bring about a fix.

Cod liver oil, vinegar rubs, and breathing in hemlock or turpentine were all medicines for TB in the mid-1800s.

Antibiotics were a significant leap forward in the treatment. In 1943, Selman Waksman, Elizabeth Bugie, and Albert Schatz created streptomycin. Waksman later got the 1952 Nobel Prize for Physiology and Medicine for this discovery.

Today, four medications are utilized to treat TB sickness: isoniazid (1951), pyrazinamide (1952), ethambutol (1961), and rifampin (1966). This four-medicated mixed drink is still the most widely recognized treatment for drug-susceptible TB.

In addition to treating this sickness, we can get dormant TB contamination to prevent the improvement of TB infection later on. Treatment for inactive TB disease can take from three to nine months.

CHAPTER 3 - HISTORY OF SMALLPOX

Origin of Smallpox

The origin of smallpox is obscure. Smallpox is thought to go back to the Egyptian Empire around the third century BCE (Before Common Era), given a smallpox—like rash found on three mummies. The soonest composed depiction of a malady that resembles smallpox showed up in China in the fourth century CE (Common Era). Early written descriptions also showed up in India in the seventh century and Asia Minor in the tenth century.

Spread of Smallpox

The worldwide spread of smallpox can be followed to the development and spread of civic establishments, investigation, and extending exchange courses throughout the hundreds of years.

Historical Highlights:

- 6th Century – Increased exchange with China and Korea brings smallpox into Japan.
- 7th Century – Arab development spreads smallpox into northern Africa, Spain, and Portugal.

- 11th Century – Crusades additionally spread smallpox in Europe.
- The 15th Century – Portuguese occupation brings smallpox into part of western Africa.
- 16th Century – European colonization and the African slave exchange import smallpox into the Caribbean and Central and South America.
- 17th Century – European colonization brings smallpox into North America.
- 18th Century – Exploration by Great Britain brings smallpox into Australia.

Early Control Efforts

Smallpox was an overwhelming sickness. Three out of each 10 individuals who got it passed on. The individuals who survived were typically left with scars, which were some of the time extremes.

One of the main strategies for controlling the spread of smallpox was the utilization of variolation. Named after the infection that causes smallpox (variola infection), variolation is the procedure by which material from smallpox wounds (pustules) was given to individuals who had never had it. This was done either by scratching the material into the armor or breathing in it through the nose. With the two sorts of variolation, individuals generally proceeded to build up the side effects related to smallpox, for example, fever and a rash. However, fewer people died from variolation than if they had procured smallpox normally.

The reason for vaccination started in 1796 when an English specialist named Edward Jenner saw that milkmaids who had gotten cowpox didn't show any symptoms of smallpox after variolation. The primary examination to test this hypothesis included milkmaid Sarah Nelmes and James Phipps, the multi-year-old child of Jenner's nursery worker. Dr. Jenner took material from a cowpox sore on Nelmes' hand and vaccinated it into Phipps' arm. Months after the fact, Jenner uncovered Phipps on various occasions to variola infection; however, Phipps never created smallpox. More analyses followed, and, in 1801, Jenner distributed his treatise "On the Origin of the Vaccine Inoculation," in which he summarized his discoveries and communicated trust that "the annihilation of smallpox, the most dreadful scourge of the human species, must be the conclusive outcome of this training."

Vaccination turned out to be broadly acknowledged and gradually replaced the practice of variolation. Sooner or later, during the 1800s (the exact time stays hazy), the infection used to make the smallpox vaccine changed from cowpox to vaccinia virus.

Hints of smallpox pustules found on the leader of a multi-year-old mummy of the Pharaoh Ramses V. Photograph courtesy of World Health Organization (WHO) Worldwide Smallpox Eradication

Edward Jenner (1749–1823). Photograph graciousness of the National Library of Medicine.

Worldwide Smallpox Eradication Program

In 1959, the World Health Organization (WHO) started a plan to free the world of smallpox. Unfortunately, this worldwide destruction battle experienced a lack of assets, workforce, and duty from countries, just as a shortage of vaccine donations. Despite their best efforts, smallpox was still far-reaching in 1966, causing normal outbreaks in numerous countries across South America, Africa, and Asia.

The Intensified Eradication Program started in 1967 with a guarantee of renewed efforts. This time, research facilities in numerous countries where smallpox happened consistently (endemic countries) had the option to create a more excellent freeze-dried vaccine. Various factors also assumed a significant job in the success of the increased efforts, including the advancement of the bifurcated needle, foundation of an observation framework to identify and research cases, and mass vaccination campaigns, to name a few.

When the Intensified Eradication Program started in 1967, smallpox had just been disposed of in North America (1952) and Europe (1953), leaving South America, Asia, and Africa (smallpox was never far-reaching in Australia). The Program gained consistent ground toward freeing the world of this illness, and by 1971 smallpox was killed from South America, trailed by Asia (1975), lastly Africa (1977).

Last Cases of Smallpox

In late 1975, Rahima Banu, a three-year-old young lady from Bangladesh, was the last person on the planet to have naturally gained variola major and the last person in Asia to have dynamic smallpox. She was isolated at home with house guards posted 24 hours every day until she was no longer infectious. A house-to-house vaccination campaign inside a 1.5-mile range of her home started quickly, and each house, public meeting area, school, and healer inside 5 miles was visited by an individual from the Smallpox Eradication Program group to guarantee the disease didn't spread. A prize was also offered to anybody for revealing a smallpox case.

Ali Maow Maalin was the last individual to have normally gained smallpox brought about by variola minor. Maalin was an emergency clinic cook in Merca, Somalia. On October 12, 1977, he went with two smallpox patients in a vehicle from the medical clinic to the local smallpox office. On October 22, he built up a fever. From the outset, he was diagnosed to have malaria and then chickenpox. He was effectively diagnosed to have smallpox by the smallpox eradication staff on October 30. Maalin was secluded and made a full recovery. Maalin kicked the bucket of jungle fever on July 22, 2013, while working in the polio eradication campaign.

Janet Parker was the last person to die of smallpox. It was 1978, and Parker was a clinical picture taker at the Birmingham University Medical School in England and worked one story over the Medical Microbiology

Department where smallpox investigation was being directed. She turned out to be sick on August 11 and built up a rash on August 15, but was not diagnosed to have smallpox until 9 days after the fact. She died on September 11, 1978. Her mom, who was giving attention to her, developed smallpox on September 7, despite having been vaccinated on August 24. An examination performed subsequently recommended that Janet Parker had been infected either using an airborne route through the clinical school building's duct system or by direct contact while visiting the microbiology corridor one floor above.

World Free of Smallpox

Right around two centuries after Jenner distributed his expectation that vaccination could annihilate smallpox, on May 8, 1980, the 33rd World Health Assembly authoritatively proclaimed the world free from this disease. Destruction of smallpox is viewed as the greatest success in international public health.

Stocks of Variola Virus

Following the eradication of smallpox, researchers and public health officials decided there was still a need to perform an investigation into utilizing the variola infection. They consented to decrease the number of research centers holding supplies of variola infection to just four areas. In 1981, the four countries that either filled in as a WHO team up focus or were effectively working with variola infection were the United States, England, Russia, and South Africa. By 1984, England and South Africa had either destroyed their stocks or moved them to other confirmed labs. There are presently just two areas where variola infection is authoritatively put away and taken care of under WHO supervision: the Centers for Disease Control and Prevention in Atlanta, Georgia, and the State Research Center of Virology and Biotechnology (VECTOR Institute) in Koltsovo, Russia.

CHAPTER 4 - PLAGUE AND BLACK DEATH (1346-1353)

The disastrous mortal disease known as the Black Death spread across Europe in the years 1346-53. Notwithstanding, the frightening name just came a few centuries after its appearance (and was presumably a mistranslation of the Latin word 'atra,' which means both 'bad' and 'dark).' Accounts and letters from the time describe the fear fashioned by the sickness. In Florence, the great Renaissance writer Petrarch was certain that they would not be accepted: 'O happy posterity, who won't experience such abysmal woe and will view our declaration as a tale.' A Florentine recorder relates that all the citizens did little else but to convey dead bodies to be covered. At each church, they dug deep pits down to the water—table, and consequently, the poor individuals who died during the night were packaged up rapidly and thrown into the pit. Toward the beginning of the day, when an enormous number of bodies were found in the pit, they took some earth and scooped it down on them. Later, others were put on them and then another layer of earth, similarly as one makes lasagna with layers of pasta and cheese.

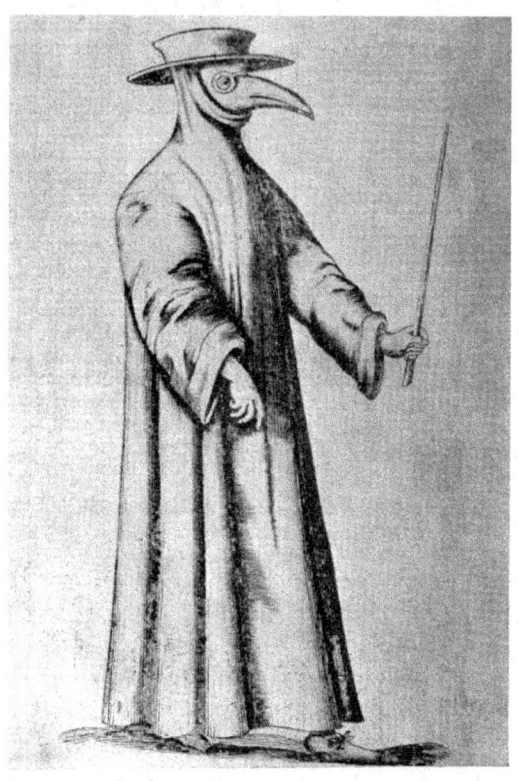

3 - *Plague doctor*[3]

The records are remarkably similar. The writer Agnolo di Tura 'the Fat' relates from his Tuscan old local that... in numerous spots in Siena, incredible pits were burrowed and heaped profound with a large number of dead. And there were additionally the individuals who were so

---

[3] **License** *Attribution 4.0 International (CC BY 4.0)* https://wellcomecollection.org/works/fguuw6k7

sparsely covered with earth that the dogs dragged them forth and ate up numerous bodies all through the city.

The tragedy was exceptional. Throughout only a couple of months, 60 percent of Florence's population died from the plague and, most likely, a similar extent in Siena. Moreover, the bare statistics, we run over significant individual disasters: Petrarch lost to the Black Death his beloved Laura to whom he wrote his well-known love sonnets; Di Tura discloses to us that 'I covered my five kids with my own hands.'

The Black Death was an epidemic of bubonic plague, a sickness brought about by the *bacterium Yersinia pestis* that prevails among wild rats where they live in great numbers and thickness. Such a region is known as a 'plague center' or a 'plague reservoir.' Plague among people emerges when rats in human residences, typically dark rodents, become tainted. The dark rat, additionally called the 'house rat' and the 'transport rat,' likes to live near individuals, the quality that makes it risky (interestingly, the brown or grey rat likes to stay away in sewers and cellars). Regularly, it takes ten to fourteen days before the plague has killed off the greater part of a contaminated rat settlement, making it hard for extraordinary quantities of insects assembled on the remaining, yet soon-dying, rats to discover new victims. Following three days of fasting, hungry rat fleas turn on people. From the chomp site, the disease channels to a lymph hub that thus swells to frame a painful bubo, regularly in the crotch, on the thigh, in an armpit, or on the neck. Thus, the bubonic name plague. The infection takes three-five days to incubate in individuals before they become sick, and in another three-five days after, in 80 percent of the cases, the victims died. Twenty-three days before the first person dies.

To turn into a plague, the disease must be spread to other rat colonies in the region and transmitted to occupants similarly. It required some investment for individuals to perceive that an awful scourge was breaking out among them and for recorders to take note of this. The timescale varies: in the wide-open, it took around forty days for the acknowledgment to daybreak; in many towns with two or three thousand inhabitants, six to seven weeks; in the urban communities with more than 10,000 inhabitants, around seven weeks, and a couple of cities with more than 100,000 occupants, as much as about two months.

Plague bacteria can break out of the buboes and be carried by the circulatory system to the lungs and cause a variety of plague that is spread by contaminated droplets from the hack of patients (pneumonic plague). However, in opposition to what is once in a while accepted, this structure isn't contracted effectively; it regularly spreads just verbosely or unexpectedly, and establishes subsequently, just a small fraction of plague cases. It presently shows up obviously that human insects and lice didn't add to the spread; at any rate, not altogether. The bloodstream of people isn't attacked by plague microorganisms from the buboes, or individuals bite the dust with scarcely any microscopic organisms in the blood that bloodsucking human parasites become inadequately infective to become infective and spread the illness: The blood of plague-infected rats contains 500-1,000 times a greater number of microbes per unit of estimation than the blood of plague-infected humans.

Significantly, the plague was spread extensively to distances by rodent insects on ships. Contaminated boat rodents would bite the dust, but their bugs would regularly survive and discover new rodents in any place they landed. In contrast to human fleas, rat fleas are adjusted to riding with their hosts; they promptly additionally swarm the dress of individuals going into influential houses and ride with them to different houses or areas. This gives plague epidemics an impossible rhythm and pace of development, with a trademark example of dispersal. The way that plague is transmitted by rat fleas means plague is a disease of the hotter seasons, which vanishes throughout the winter, or if nothing else, loses a large portion of their powers of spread.

The peculiar seasonal pattern of plague has been watched all over the place and is a systematic component of the spread of the Black Death. In the plague history of Norway, from the Black Death in 1348-49 to the last flare-ups in 1654, involving more than thirty floods of plague, there was never a winter epidemic of plague. Plague is different from airborne contagious diseases, which are spread directly between individuals by beads: these thrive in cold weather.

It used to be felt that the Black Death started in China, but new research shows that it started in the spring of 1346 in the steppe district, where a plague store extends from the northwestern shores of the Caspian Sea into southern Russia. Individuals every so often contract plague there even today. Two contemporary chroniclers identify the estuary of the stream Don, where it streams into the Sea of Azov as the area of the first flare-up, yet this could be a mere rumor, and it is possible that it began somewhere else; maybe in the area of the estuary of the waterway Volga on the Caspian Sea. At that point, this area was under the standard of the Mongol khanate of the Golden Horde. A few decades sooner, the Mongol khanate had changed over to Islam, and the presence of Christians or exchange with them was never again tolerated. Accordingly, the Silk Road band courses among China and Europe were cut off. For a similar reason, the Black Death didn't spread from the east through Russia towards Western Europe but stopped abruptly on the Mongol outskirt with the Russian areas. Thus, Russia, which may have become the Black Death's first European success, in reality, was its last, and was attacked by the infection not from the east but from the west. The plague, in reality, started with an attack that the Mongols launched on the Italian vendors' last trading station the district, Kaffa (today Feodosiya) in the Crimea. In the harvest time of 1346, plague broke out among the besiegers and, from them, entered into the town. When spring showed up, the Italians fled on their boats. And the Black Death slipped unnoticed and sailed with them.

The extent of the contagious power of the Black Death has been practically mystifying. The focal clarification exists in the characteristic features of medieval society in a powerful period of modernization proclaiming the change from a medieval to early current European society. Early mechanical market-financial and free enterprise improvements had advanced more than is regularly expected, particularly in northern Italy and Flanders. New, bigger kinds of the ship carried great quantities of products over broad exchange arrangement that connected Venice and Genoa with Constantinople and the Crimea, Alexandria, and Tunis, London and Bruges. In London and Bruges, the Italian trading system was connected to the bustling delivery lines of the German Hanseatic League in the Nordic nations and the Baltic area, with huge expansive bellied boats called machine gear-pieces. This system for the long-separation exchange was supplemented by a web of lively short and medium-distance trade that bound together populations everywhere throughout the Old World.

As effectively noticed, the pace of spread slowed strongly during the winter and halted totally in mountain areas, for example, the Alps and the northern pieces of Europe. However, the Black Death regularly quickly settled at least two fronts and vanquished nations by progressing from different quarters.

Italian boats from Kaffa showed up in Constantinople in May 1347 with the Black Death ready. The epidemic broke loose at the beginning of July. In North Africa and the Middle East, it began around September first, having shown up in Alexandria with transport from Constantinople. It's spread from Constantinople to European Mediterranean business center points, and additionally began in the pre-winter of 1347. It arrived at Marseilles by about the second seven-day stretch of September, presumably with a boat from the city. At that point, the Italian traders seem to have left Constantinople a while later and showed up in the places where they grew up of Genoa and Venice with plague ready, sometime in November. On their way home, ships from Genoa additionally sullied Florence's seaport city of Pisa. The spread out of Pisa is described by various metastatic leaps. These extraordinary business urban communities additionally worked as bridgeheads from where the disease conquered Europe.

In transit to Spain, the Black Death additionally struck out from the city of Narbonne north-westwards along the principal street to the business focus of Bordeaux on the Atlantic coast, which before the end of March had become a basic new focal point of spread. Around April twentieth, a boat from Bordeaux probably showed up in La Coruña in northwestern Spain; a long time later, another boat from that point let free the plague in Navarre in northeastern Spain. Along these lines, two northern plague fronts were opened under two months after the disease had invaded southern Spain.

The early arrival of the Black Death in England and the quick spread to its southeastern regions shaped a great part of the example of spread in Northern Europe. The plague more likely than not showed up in Oslo in the harvest time of 1348 and probably accompanied a boat from southeastern England, which had vivacious business contacts with Norway. The outbreak of the Black Death in Norway occurred before the disease had figured out how to penetrate southern Germany, again delineating the great importance of transportation by transport and the overall gradualness of spread via land. The flare-up in Oslo was before long stopped by the coming of winter climate, yet it broke out again in the late winter. Before long, it spread out of Oslo along the fundamental streets inland and on the two sides of the Oslofjord. Another independent introduction of contagion happened toward the beginning of July 1349 in the town of Bergen; it showed up in a boat from England, most likely from King's Lynn. The opening of the subsequent plague front was the explanation that all Norway could be conquered throughout 1349. It disappeared totally with the winter approaches, and the last victims passed on at the turn of the year.

CHAPTER 5 - CHOLERA

Cholera, brought about by the microorganism *Vibrio cholerae*, is uncommon in the United States and other industrialized countries. However, globally, cholera cases have expanded consistently since 2005, and the disease, despite everything, happens in numerous spots, including Africa, Southeast Asia, and Haiti. CDC reacts to cholera episodes worldwide utilizing its Global Water, Sanitation, and Hygiene (WASH) expertise.

Cholera can be dangerous, yet it is easily prevented and treated. Travelers, public health, clinical experts, and outbreak responders ought to know about areas with high paces of cholera, know how the sickness spreads, and what to do to prevent it.

Illness & Symptoms

Cholera is an intense, diarrheal illness brought about by disease of the digestive tract with the bacterium, *Vibrio cholerae* and is spread by the ingestion of contaminated nourishment or water. The infection is frequently mellow or without side effects; however, some of the time, it tends to be extreme and threatening.

Around one of every ten (5-10%) of infected people will have extreme cholera, which in the early stages includes:

- Profuse watery diarrhea, now and then depicted as "rice-water stools"
- Vomiting
- Rapid pulse
- Loss of skin flexibility
- Dry mucous films
- Low circulatory strain
- Thirst
- Muscle cramps
- Restlessness or irritability

People with serious cholera can create intense renal failure, extreme electrolyte imbalances, and coma. If untreated, extreme drying out can quickly lead to shock and death in hours.

Profuse diarrhea produced by cholera patients contains a lot of infectious *Vibrio cholerae* microorganisms that can infect others whenever ingested, and when these microbes defile water or nourishment, it will lead to extra diseases. Dispose of human waste appropriately will prevent the spread of cholera.

People thinking about cholera patients can avoid acquiring disease by washing their hands in the wake of contacting whatever may be contaminated and properly disposing of infected things and human waste.

Infected people, when treated quickly, can recover rapidly, and there are regularly no long-term outcomes. People with cholera don't become transporters of the disease after they recoup, yet can be re-infected if exposed again.

Sources of Infection and Risk Factors

Cholera is an intense intestinal disease-causing profuse watery diarrhea, vomiting, circulatory breakdown, and stunning. Numerous infections are related to milder runs or with no indications by any means. Whenever left untreated, half of the extreme cholera cases can be fatal.

Diagnosis and Detection

It is practically difficult to recognize a single patient with cholera from a patient infected by another pathogen that causes acute watery diarrhea without a feces test. A survey of clinical features of various patients who are part of a suspected outbreak of acute watery diarrhea can help distinguish cholera given the fast spread of the illness.

While the management of patients with acute watery diarrhea is comparative, it is essential to identify cholera as a result of the potential for a broad outbreak.

The Most Effective Method to Diagnose

Isolation and identification proof of *Vibrio cholerae* serogroup O1 or O139 by a culture of a stool sample remains the highest quality level for the research center diagnosis of cholera.

Cary Blair media is perfect for transport, and the specific thiosulfate–citrate–bile salts agar (TCBS) is perfect for isolation and identification. Reagents for sero-grouping *Vibrio cholerae* isolates are available in all state well-being office research centers in the U.S. Economically available quick test units are valuable in epidemic settings. However, they don't provide the allowance for antibiotic susceptibility testing and subtyping and ought not to be utilized for routine diagnosis.

In numerous countries where cholera isn't exceptional, and access to diagnostic laboratory testing is difficult, WHO suggests the following clinical definition be utilized for suspected cholera cases.

Suspected Cholera Case

- In areas where a cholera flare-up has not been announced: Any patient 2 years of age or more established giving with acute watery diarrhea and extreme lack of hydration or dying from acute watery diarrhea.
- In areas where a cholera flare-up is announced: any individual giving or passing on from acute watery diarrhea.

WHO additionally prescribes the following definition for confirmed cholera cases?

Confirmed Cholera Case

A suspected case with *Vibrio cholerae* O1 or O139 confirmed by culture or PCR and, in nations where cholera is absent or has been wiped out, the *Vibrio cholerae* O1 or O139 strain is shown to be toxigenic.

Quick Tests

In areas with restricted or no research center testing, the Crystal® VC dipstick quick test can give an early admonition to public health officials that an outbreak of cholera is happening. Nonetheless, the precision and accuracy of this test aren't ideal. In this way, it is suggested that fecal examples that test positive for *V. cholerae* O1 as well as O139 by the Crystal® VC dipstick consistently be confirmed utilizing customary culture-based strategies reasonable for the isolation and identification proof of *V. cholerae*.

Treatment

Most people infected with the cholera bacterium have mellow loose bowels or no side effects by any means. Just a little proportion, around 5-10% of people infected with *Vibrio cholerae* O1 may have an illness requiring treatment at a health center. Cholera patients ought to be assessed and treated rapidly. With appropriate treatment, even seriously sick patients can be saved.

Cholera Treatments

- **Rehydration treatment**, which means brief reclamation of lost liquids and salts through rehydration treatment, is the essential objective of treatment.
- **Antibiotic treatment**, which reduces fluid requirements and duration of disease, is indicated for extreme instances of cholera.

- **Zinc treatment** has additionally been observed to help improve cholera side effects in kids.

CHAPTER 6 - SPANISH INFLUENZA

(1918-20)

Over the most recent 150 years, the world has seen a remarkable improvement in health. The visualization shows that in numerous nations' futures, the normal life expectancy multiplied from around 40 years or less to over 80 years. This was not only an achievement over these countries; the future has multiplied in all regions of the world.

What additionally stands apart is how unexpected and damning negative well-being occasions can be. Most striking is the huge, unexpected decrease of the future in 1918, brought about by a strangely savage flu pandemic that got known as the 'Spanish flu.'

To understand the reality of the future declining, so suddenly, one needs to understand what it measures. Period future is the exact name for this measure. Just take a look at the mortality design in one specific year and then it captures this snapshot of population health as the normal time of death of a hypothetical cohort of individuals for which that year's mortality example would stay consistent all through their whole lifetimes. Period future is a proportion of the population's health in one year.

History of 1918 Flu Pandemic (Española)

The 1918 flu pandemic was the most extreme in ongoing history. It was brought about by an H1N1 infection with qualities of avian origin. Although there isn't general agreement in regards to where the infection began, it spread overall during 1918-1919. In the United States, it was first identified in military staff in spring 1918.

It is assessed that 500 million individuals or 33% of the total population got infected with this infection. The number of deaths was evaluated to be in any event 50 million worldwide, with around 675,000 happenings in the United States. Mortality was high in individuals more youthful than 5 years of age, 20-40 years of age, and 65 years and more. The high mortality in healthy people, incorporating those in the 20-multiyear age gathering, was a novel component of this pandemic.

While the 1918 H1N1 infection has been synthesized and evaluated, the properties that made it so annihilating are not surely known. With no vaccine to ensure against flu disease and no anti-toxins to treat optional bacterial infections that can be related to flu infections, control efforts overall were restricted to non-pharmaceutical mediations like disconnection, isolation, great individual cleanliness, utilization of disinfectants, and impediments of open social occasions, which were applied unevenly.

This flu outbreak wasn't confined to Spain, and it didn't start there; the scourge began in New York because of proof of a pre-pandemic rush of the infection in that city).

In any case, it was accordingly named because Spain was nonpartisan in the First World War (1914-18), which meant it was allowed to investigate the seriousness of the pandemic, while countries that were fighting tried to stifle information about how the flu affected their populace to keep up confidence and not appear weakened in the eyes of the enemies.

The flu episode began in the Northern Hemisphere in the spring of 1918. The infection spread quickly and inevitably arrived at all places of the world: the plague turned into a pandemic.

Indeed, even in a significantly less-associated world, the infection, in the long run, arrived at incredibly remote places, for example, the Alaskan wild and Samoa in the Pacific islands.

While top mortality was come to in 1918, the pandemic didn't end until two years after the fact in late 1920.

The Global Death Count of the Flu Today

To have a setting for the severity of influenza pandemics, it may be useful to realize the death check of a run of the mill influenza season. Current estimates for the yearly number of deaths from the flu are around 400,000 deaths each year—a normal of 389,000 with a vulnerability run 294,000 from 518,000.

This means, as of late, seasonal influenza was liable for the demise of 0.0052% of the total population – one individual out of 18,750. Even in comparison with the low measure for the passing check of Spanish influenza (17.4 million), this pandemic, over a century back, caused a death rate that was 182 - times higher than the present pattern.

Note: Shown is a period future during childbirth, the normal number of years an infant would live if the example of mortality in the given year were to remain the same throughout its life.

Worldwide Deaths of the Spanish Flu

A few research groups have taken a shot at the tough issue of remaking the global health impact of the pandemic. There is currently a great deal of inconsistency in these varieties, and keeping in mind that the scholarly discussions proceed with the scope of evaluations gives us an understanding of the severity of the occasion.

The visualization here shows the available estimates from the distinctive research distribution talked about in the following:

Patterson and Pyle (1991) evaluated that somewhere in the range of 24.7 and 39.3 million died from the pandemic.

The broadly referred to concentrate by Johnson and Mueller (2002) shows up at a lot higher estimate of 50 million worldwide deaths. In any case, the authors recommend this could be an underestimation and that the genuine death toll was as high as 100 million.

The later examination by Spreeuwenberg et al. (2018) presumed that prior appraisals have been excessively high. Their estimate is 17.4 million deaths; worldwide death rate.

How do these estimates compare to the size of the total population at that point? How enormous was the number that died in the pandemic?

Assessments recommend that the total populace in 1918 was 1.8 billion.

Given this, the low gauge of 17.4 million deaths, Spanish influenza, murdered nearly 1% (0.95%) of the world population.

If we depend on the gauge of 50 million deaths distributed by Johnson and Mueller, it suggests that Spanish influenza murdered 2.7% of the total population. What's more, if it was in certainty higher at 100 million as these authors recommend, then the worldwide death rate would have been 5.4%.

The total population was developed by around 13 million consistently; this presupposes that the time of the Spanish influenza was likely the last time in history when the total population was declining.

Other Large Influenza Pandemics

The Spanish influenza pandemic was the biggest, yet by all accounts, not the only huge late flu pandemic. Two decades before Spanish influenza, the Russian influenza pandemic (1889-1894) is accepted to have murdered 1 million people.

Evaluations for the death toll of the "Asian Flu" (1957-1958) differ somewhere in the range of 1.5 and 4 million. The estimate was 1.5 million, while Michaelis et al. (2009) published an estimate of 2–4 million.

As per a WHO production, the "Hong Kong Flu" (1968-1969) killed somewhere in the range of 1 and 4 million people. Michaelis et al. (2009) published a lower estimate of 1–2 million.

The Russian Flu pandemic of 1977-78 was brought about by the equivalent H1N1 infection that caused Spanish influenza. As per Michaelis et al. (2009), around 700,000 died worldwide.

What turns out to be obvious from this review are two things: flu pandemics are not uncommon, yet the Spanish influenza of 1918 was by a long shot the most destroying flu pandemic in written history.

The Effect of the Spanish Influenza Pandemic on Various Age Groups

This last representation shows the feature in England and Wales by age. The red line shows the feature for a newborn, with the rainbow-colored lines above demonstrating to what extent an individual could hope to live once they had arrived at that given, older age. The light green line, for instance, speaks to the future for youngsters who had arrived at age 10.

It shows that the future expanded at all ages, which implies that the frequently heard assertion that the future 'just' expanded because youngster mortality declined isn't valid. This long-term rise of life expectancy at all ages is the focal point of this; going with the content here.

As for the effect of the Spanish flu, it is striking that the perception shows that the pandemic had almost no effect on older people. While the future during childbirth and at young ages declined by over ten years, the future of 60- and 70-year olds saw no change. This is inconsistent with what we would expect: Older populations tend to be generally vulnerable to flu outbreaks and respiratory infections. If we take a look at mortality for both lower respiratory diseases (pneumonia) and upper respiratory infections today, death rates are most noteworthy for the individuals who are 70 years and older.

One motivation behind why this pandemic was so destructive was that youngsters represented a large share of the population.

For what reason were more seasoned individuals so strong to the 1918 pandemic? The examination writing recommends this was the situation because more seasoned individuals had survived a prior influenza outbreak – the as of now talked about 'Russian flu pandemic' of 1889–90 — which gave the individuals who survived it some resistance for the later outbreak of the Spanish flu.

The prior 1889–90 pandemic may have given the older population some insusceptibility, yet it was a damaging occasion in itself. As indicated by Smith, 132,000 individuals died in England, Wales, and Ireland alone.

We've also observed that during Spanish influenza, and numerous nations attempted to smother any data about the flu outbreak. Today the sharing of information, research, and news are surely not great but altogether different and considerably more open than previously.

However, the facts demonstrate that the present reality is vastly improved comparatively. In 1918, it was railways and steamships that dominated the world. Today planes can convey individuals and infections to numerous edges of the world in a very short time.

Differences in health frameworks and foundation additionally matter. Spanish influenza hit the world in the prior days anti-toxins were designed, and numerous deaths, maybe most, were not brought about by the flu infection itself, yet by auxiliary bacterial diseases. During Spanish influenza, "most of the deaths... likely came about legitimately from optional bacterial pneumonia brought about by regular upper respiratory–tract bacteria."

Furthermore, health frameworks were extraordinary, yet additionally, the health and living states of the worldwide population. The year 1918 hit a total population of which a huge offer was incredibly poor. In essence, enormous portions of the population were undernourished; in many parts of the world, the populaces lived in unforeseen weakness, congestion, and poor sanitation; low hygiene standards were normal. Also, the populaces in numerous pieces of the world were debilitated by a worldwide war. Public resources were little, and numerous nations had quite recently spent huge portions of their assets on the war.

While the greater part of the world is much richer and healthier now, the worry today also is that it is the poorest people that will be hit hardest by the new virus.

These distinctions propose that one ought to be cautious in drawing exercises from the outbreak a century ago.

In any case, Spanish influenza reminds us exactly how enormous the effect of a pandemic can be, even in nations that had just been successful in improving population health. Another pathogen can make horrible annihilations and lead to the death of millions. Thus Spanish influenza has been referred to as a notice and as inspiration to get ready for enormous pandemic flare-ups, which have been viewed as likely by numerous analysts. Justinian's Plague (541-542 CE)

During the rule of the head Justinian I (527-565 CE), one of the worst outbreaks of the plague occurred, killing a large number of individuals. The plague showed up in Constantinople in 542 CE, close to 12 months after the malady originally showed up in the external regions of the empire. The outbreak kept on clearing all through the

Mediterranean world for an additional 225 years, and at last, disappearing in 750 CE.

Plague Origination and Transmission

Starting in China and upper east India, the plague (*Yersinia pestis*) was carried to the Great Lakes district of Africa through overland and ocean exchange courses. The purpose of origin for Justinian's plague was Egypt. The Byzantine historian Procopius of Caesarea (500-565 CE) identified the start of the plague in Pelusium on the Nile River's northern and eastern shores. As indicated by Wendy Orent, writer of Plague, the infection spread in two ways: north to Alexandria and east to Palestine.

The method for transmission of the plague was the black rat (Rattus rattus), which went on the grain ships and trucks sent to Constantinople as a tribute. North Africa, in the eighth century CE, was the primary source of grain for the empire, alongside various wares including paper, oil, ivory, and slaves. Put away in vast warehouses, and the grain gave an ideal rearing ground to the bugs and rodents, urgent to the transmission of plague. William Rosen, in Justinian's Flea, fights that while rats are known to eat pretty much anything (counting vegetable issue and little animals), the grain is their preferred dinner. Rosen further sees that rats, for the most part, don't travel more than 200 meters from their origination through the span of their lifetimes. In any case, once onboard the grain boats and carts, the rats were carried throughout the empire.

As indicated by historian Colin Barras, Procopius recorded the climatic changes occurring in southern Italy during the period: unusual incidents of snow and frost in the amidst summer, below normal temperatures, and a reduction of daylight. So started a decades-in length frosty spell joined by social interruptions, war, and the main recorded outbreak of the plague. The colder than normal climate influenced crop harvests, leading to food deficiencies that brought about the developments of individuals all through the district. Accompanying these reluctant migrants were plague-infected, flea-ridden rats. Chilly, worn out, hungry individuals in a hurry, joined with disease and illness amidst the fighting, just as an expanded rat population carrying a highly infectious disease, made the ideal conditions for a pestilence. Also, what a scourge it would be: named after the Byzantine ruler Justinian I (482-565 CE; emperorship 527-565 CE), Justinian's plague influenced a large portion of the number of inhabitants in Europe.

Kinds of Plague and Symptoms

In the light of DNA investigation of bones found in graves, the sort of plague that struck the Byzantine Empire during the rule of Justinian was bubonic (*Yersinia pestis*). However, it was truly likely that the other two kinds of plague, pneumonic and septicemic, were also present. It was additionally bubonic plague that would devastate the fourteenth century CE Europe (also called the Black Death), killing as much as 50 million individuals or almost a large portion of the whole population of the continent. A plague was not new to history, even in the hour of Justinian. Wendy Orent proposes that the principal recorded record of bubonic plague is told in the Old Testament in the tale of the Philistines who took the Ark of the Covenant from the Israelites and surrendered to "swellings."

Procopius, in his Secret History, describes the victims as experiencing delusions, nightmares, fevers, and swellings in the groin, armpits, and behind their ears. Procopius describes that, while a few sufferers lapsed into a trance-like state, others turned out to be exceptionally unusual. Numerous victims languished over days before death, while others passed on very quickly after the beginning of the manifestations. Procopius' depiction of the disease more likely than not confirms the nearness of bubonic plague as the fundamental guilty party of the outbreak. He laid the blame for the outbreak on the head, pronouncing Justinian to be either a fallen angel or that the sovereign was being rebuffed by God for his evil ways.

CHAPTER 7 - THE SPREAD OF THE PLAGUE THROUGH THE BYZANTINE EMPIRE

War and exchanges encouraged the spread of the sickness all through the Byzantine Empire. Justinian spent the early long periods of his reign defeating a variety of enemies: struggling with Ostrogoth for command over Italy; struggling Vandals and Berbers for control in North Africa; and struggling off Franks, Slavs, Avars, and other savage clans occupied with attacks against the empire. History specialists have recommended that officers and the inventory trains supporting their military efforts, acting as the means for the rodents and insects carrying the plague. By 542 CE, Justinian had re-conquered a large portion of his realm at the same time as when Wendy Orent brings up harmony, success, and trade, which additionally gave proper conditions to encouraging a plague outbreak. Constantinople, the political capital of the eastern Roman Empire, served as the focal point of business exchange for the empire. The capital's area along the Black and Aegean oceans made it the ideal crossroads for exchange courses from China, the

Middle East, and North Africa. Where exchange and business went, so went rats, insects, and the plague.

Wendy Orent accounts for the course of the sickness. Following the built-up exchange courses of the realm, the plague moved from Ethiopia to Egypt and then all through the Mediterranean region. The disease penetrated neither northern Europe nor the open country, proposing that black rat was the essential bearer of the tainted insect as the rats held near the ports and ships. The episode kept going around for months in Constantinople; however, would keep on persevering for generally the following three centuries, with the last flare-up detailed in 750 CE. There would not be any more huge scope outbreaks of the plague until the fourteenth century CE Black Death scene.

The plague was broad to such an extent that nobody was protected; even the ruler came down with the sickness; however, he didn't die. Dead bodies littered the streets of the capital. Justinian requested soldiers to aid the removal of the dead. When the memorial parks and tombs were filled, burial pits and channels were burrowed to deal with the flood. Bodies were disposed of in buildings, dumped into the ocean, and set on boats for burials at sea. Furthermore, it was not only human beings who were infected; creatures of various types, including felines and hounds, died and required legitimate removal.

Plague Treatment

When infected, individuals had two strategies: treatment by clinical workforce or home remedies. William Rosen distinguishes the clinical workforce as essentially prepared doctors. A considerable lot of the doctors were occupied with a four-year course of study instructed by prepared specialists (iastrophists) at Alexandria, which at that point was the head place for clinical training. The training got by the understudies focused on the lessons of the Greek doctor Galen (129-217 CE), who was affected in his understanding of the disease by the idea of humorism. This clinical framework depended on the treatment of disease dependent on bodily fluids, known as "senses of humor."

Lacking access to one of the kinds of doctors, private individuals frequently went for home cures. Rosen recognizes different methodologies that individuals took towards treating the plague, including cold-water showers, powders "favored" by holy people, enchantment ornaments and rings, and different medications, particularly alkaloids. Failing all the past ways to deal with treatment, individuals went to medical clinics or ended up subject to isolation. The people who survived were ascribed, as per Rosen, with "favorable fortune, strong underlying health, and a positive immune system."

Impacts on the Byzantine Empire

The plague scene added to a debilitating of the Byzantine Empire in political and economical manners. As the infection spread all through the Mediterranean world, the realm's capacity to oppose its adversaries debilitated. By 568 CE, the Lombard effectively attacked northern Italy and defeated the little Byzantine battalion, leading to the fracturing of the Italian peninsula, which stayed isolated and split until re-unification in the nineteenth century CE. In the Roman areas of North Africa and the Near East, the realm couldn't stem the encroachment of Arabs. The reduced size and the inability of the Byzantine armed force to oppose outside powers was to a great extent because of its failure to select and prepare new volunteers for the spread of disease and death. The decline in the population not just affected the military and the empire's protection, but also the financial and regulatory structures of the empire began to collapse or disappear.

Exchange all through the empire got disturbed. Specifically, the farming segment was devastated. Fewer individuals meant fewer ranchers who created less grain, making costs take off and charge incomes to decrease. The close to falling off the financial framework didn't prevent Justinian from requesting a similar degree of assessment from his decimated population. On his assurance to reproduce the previous Mayor of the Roman Empire, the sovereign kept on taking up arms against the Goths in Italy and the Vandals at Carthage, in case his empire disintegrate. The head also stayed focused on a progression of openwork, and church development extends in the capital, including the structure of the Hagia Sophia.

Procopius reported in his Secret History of almost 10,000 deaths for every day afflicting Constantinople. His exactness has been addressed by present-day historians who estimate 5,000 deaths for each day in the capital city. In any case, 20-40% of the occupants of Constantinople would, in the end, die from the disease. All through the remainder of the empire, about 25% of the population died, with the estimates extending from 25-50 million people in total.

CHAPTER 8 - HONG KONG FLU (1968 INFLUENZA PANDEMIC)

The 1968 flu pandemic (the "Hong Kong influenza") was a classification 2 influenza pandemic, whose outbreak in 1968 and 1969 killed an expected one million individuals around the world. Hong Kong influenza was one of the famous flu pandemics in history. It was brought about by an H3N2 strain of the flu. An infection dropped from H2N2 through an antigenic move, a genetic process wherein qualities from various subtypes re-assorted to frame another infection. The Hong Kong Flu (1968 pandemic flu) H3N2 Hemagglutinin (HA) proteins and antibodies were the primary research devices for this flu pandemic.

Hong Kong Flu History

The primary record of the episode in Hong Kong showed up on 13 July 1968. Before the finish of July 1968, broad outbreaks were accounted for in Vietnam and Singapore. Despite the casualty of the 1957 Asian flu in China, little improvement had been made concerning the treatment of such pandemics. The Times paper was the primary source to sound alarmed concerning this new possible pandemic.

By September 1968, this season's cold virus arrived in India, Philippines, northern Australia, and Europe. That equivalent month, the infection entered California from returning Vietnam War troops but didn't get far-reaching in the US until December 1968. It would arrive in Japan, Africa, and South America by 1969. The outbreak in Hong Kong, where density is around 500 individuals for each section of land, arrived with most extreme force in about fourteen days, lasting a month and a half altogether from July to December 1968. Anyway, overall deaths from this infection peaked much later, in December 1968 and January 1969. At that point, public health warnings and infection portrayals were given in the logical and medical journals.

A similar infection reoccurred the next years: after a year, in late 1969 and mid-1970, and 1972.

America wasn't immune either. The infection entered California using troops coming back from the Vietnam War but didn't get spread there until December 1968.

Around the world, the deaths from Hong Kong influenza crested in December 1968 and January 1969.

While the strain had a moderately low death rate (the 1918-19 Spanish influenza pandemic, for instance, killed between 25 million and 50 million), it was exceptionally infectious. Symptoms kept going on for four to five days, and at times as long as about fourteen days. The infection caused upper respiratory symptoms regular of flu, including chills, fever, muscle pain, and weakness.

The next day, July 25, the Post investigated the cost this season's cold virus was taking on open utilities and industry.

"Worst hit among the public utilities were the Hong Kong Telephone Co, and China Light and Power. Two hundred of 300 laborers of each organization were infected," the paper revealed.

And, it wasn't just human life that was affected.

On May 1, 1969, the Post published a story by universal news organization UPI with the attention-grabbing headline "EVEN WHALES CATCH HK FLU." The report said three whales – Shamu, Kilroy and Ramu — at Sea World in the Californian city of San Diego had contracted Hong Kong influenza and must be dosed with anti-infection pills disguised in mackerel. (Ramu was the hardest hit, and was getting 375 pills like clockwork, as per his veterinary specialist, Dr. David Kenney.)

January 1970, a report in The New York Times said: "researchers speculate that at any rate, three of the ongoing pandemics of flu started in mainland China." A selection from the story peruses: Dr. Chang Wai-kwan of Hong Kong's Queen Mary Hospital was cited as telling an international conference: "The Asian influenza of 1957 began in the focal terrain of the People's Republic of China, and the pestilence of 1968 could have originated from a similar source."

China, instead of Spain, was also now accepted to have been the source of the deadliest twentieth-century influenza pandemic, the report said.

"The incredible pandemic of 1918-1919, wrongly called Spanish influenza, showed up first in quite a while in China," an ongoing review in the British Medical Journal said. "The plague of 1889, which moved from the depths of Russia westbound across Europe, could likewise have started in China, Dr. Alexander D. Langmuir, boss disease transmission specialist at the [US] National Communicable Disease Center in Atlanta, said."

A World Health Organization Report

The study of disease transmission of Hong Kong Influenza, from 1969, credits Hong Kong by participating rapidly and effectively so "they could seclude the strain and build up an antibody."

"So far as the isolation and characterization of the infection were concerned, the program satisfied its goal and, gratitude to the efforts of the national reference community in Hong Kong and the two global focuses. The strain was secluded, distributed and identified to antibody makers with all conceivable speed," the report said. "It is hard to imagine conditions in which the interim from the appearance of examples in a national flu community to the characterization and appropriation of the strain could be shortened."

And keeping in mind that propels in medication and technology means fewer deaths, regular flu can even now be lethal. Simply a week ago, a nine-year-old young lady died in Hong Kong in the wake of getting seasonal influenza, the third such demise revealed in 2018. (She had other chronic illnesses.)

Hong Kong influenza is, by all accounts, not the only deadly disease outbreak to have hit the city. In 1997, 18 individuals were infected, and six passed on when H5N1 bird flu initially bounced the species obstruction from poultry to individuals. In late December of that year, the service requested the slaughter of 1.3 million chickens in an offer to stop the spread of the infection.

In 2009, Hong Kong recorded the main instance of swine influenza in Asia. Be that as it may, nothing hit the city harder than severe acute respiratory syndrome (Sars) in 2003, which contaminated 1,755 individuals in Hong Kong and killed 299 of them.

CHAPTER 9 - HIV AND AIDS

The (AIDS) scourge has substantially affected the health and economy of numerous countries. Since the principal AIDS cases were accounted for in the United States in June 1981, the number of cases and deaths among people with AIDS expanded quickly during the 1980s, followed by considerable decreases in new cases and deaths in the late 1990s. This report depicts the adjustments in the attributes of people with AIDS since 1981. The best effect of the pandemic is among men who engage in sexual relations with men (MSM) and among racial/ethnic minorities, with increments in the number of cases among ladies and of cases credited to hetero transmission. The quantity of people living with AIDS has expanded as deaths have declined. Controlling the plague requires continued prevention programs in these at-risk networks, especially programs focusing on MSM, ladies, and injection drug users.

CDC broke down revealed AIDS cases from 1981 through 2000 from the 50 states, District of Columbia, and U.S. regions. Prevalence by sex, age, race/ethnicity, area, and crucial status (living or deceased) were figured more than four time-spans relating to changes in the AIDS case definition and the introduction of effective combination antiretroviral treatment. Patterns in evaluated AIDS findings and deaths of people with AIDS were balanced for revealing differences dependent on the number of cases reported to CDC through June 2000, and for anticipated reclassification of cases initially announced without human immunodeficiency virus (HIV) disease hazard data. Assessed AIDS predominance was determined as the combined occurrence of AIDS less total deaths balanced for revealing postponements.

As of December 31, 2000, 774,467 people had been accounted for with AIDS in the United States; 448,060 of these had died; 3542 people had obscure crucial status. The quantity of people living with AIDS (322,865) is the most elevated at any point detailed. Of these, 79% were men, 61% were dark or Hispanic, and 41% were infected through male-to-male sex. Of the AIDS cases, around 33% were accounted for during 1981 –1992, 1993 – 1995, and 1996 – 2000.

Helps frequency expanded quickly through the 1980s, topped in the mid-1990s, and then declined. The peak of new diagnoses was related to the extension of the AIDS surveillance case definition in 1993. Starting in 1996, sharp declines were accounted for in AIDS occurrence and deaths. From 1998 through June 2000, AIDS rate and deaths leveled off, and AIDS prevalence kept on expanding. All through the plague, around 85% of people determined to have AIDS were aged 20 – 49 years.

In the mid-1980s, most AIDS cases happened among whites. However, cases among blacks expanded consistently, and by 1996, a larger number of cases happened among blacks than some other racial/ethnic population. Cases among Hispanics, Asians/Pacific Islanders, and American Indians/Alaska Natives have increased also.

Male-to-male sex has been the most well-known method of introduction among people reported with AIDS (46%), trailed by infusion medication use (25%), and hetero contact (11%). The rate of AIDS expanded quickly in every one of the three of these risk categories through the mid-1990s, but, since 1996, decreases in new AIDS cases have been higher among MSM and injection drug users than among people revealed through heterosexual contact.

Almost all transmission of HIV through transfusion of blood or blood items happened before the screening of the blood supply for HIV neutralizer was started in 1985. The number of people detailed with AIDS who were revealed through blood transfusions was 284 in 2000, down from a peak of 1098 in 1993. The quantity of perinatally procured AIDS cases peaked in 1992 (901 cases), followed by a sharp decline through December 1999. In 1999, 144 instances of perinatally gained AIDS were diagnosed.

On June 5, 1981, MMWR distributed a report of *Pneumocystis carinii* pneumonia in five previously healthy young men in Los Angeles, California. These cases were later perceived as the first reported cases of acquired immunodeficiency syndrome (AIDS) in the United States. Since that time, this disease has gotten one of the best general health challenges, both broadly and all-inclusive. Human immunodeficiency virus (HIV) and AIDS have killed more than 22 million people around the world, remembering more than 500,000 people in the United States.

In 2006, more than 1 million people were living with HIV/AIDS in the United States, and an expected 40,000 new HIV diseases are required to happen this year. Since the start of the epidemic, countless persons and organizations, inside and outside of government, have activated to forestall and treat this disease. These efforts have been upgraded by the dedication and association of those living with HIV/AIDS. At this achievement denoting the 25th year of AIDS, one approach to remember those people who have died and the individuals who have been influenced by this scourge is to quicken the advancement of measures for preventing HIV transmission.

Successes in HIV Prevention

CDC's overarching HIV prevention objective is to lessen the quantity of new HIV diseases and to dispense with racial and ethnic disparities by the advancement of HIV directing, testing, and referral and by empowering HIV prevention among the two people living with HIV and those at high threat for getting the infection.

The reduction in mother-to-child (perinatal) HIV transmission is a public health achievement in HIV prevention in the United States. The number of newborn children infected with HIV through perinatal transmission has reduced from 1,650 during the ahead of schedule to mid-1990s to 144 – 236 in all 2002. This decline is ascribed to numerous interventions, including routine willful HIV testing of pregnant ladies, the utilization of fast HIV tests at delivery for ladies of obscure HIV status, and the utilization of antiretroviral treatment of HIV-positive ladies during pregnancy and by newborn children after birth.

Across the board, availability and utilization of demonstrative and screening tests for HIV disease to advance individual information on HIV serostatus and to guarantee the safety of the country's blood supply has been another achievement. Since the mid-1980s, blood giver screening techniques and testing innovation have consistently improved; today, with nucleic acid testing, the risk for HIV transmission is evaluated at as low as one for every 2 million blood gifts. Far-reaching HIV testing advancement and take-up have come about in around half of people aged 15 – 44 years in the United States announcing that they have had an HIV test, with a high extent of those at expanded hazard (e.g., men who have sex with men [MSM] and sedate infusion clients) detailing having an HIV test during the former year.

National HIV anticipation activities have been supported by HIV counteraction projects of state and local health departments, community-based organizations, and different partners. Counteraction intercessions, including drug treatment programs, peer effort, and risk decrease, have added to a consistent decrease in new HIV/AIDS analysis among sedate infusion clients in 35 regions with HIV announcing, from an expected 8,048 in 2001 to 5,962 in 2004. Another anticipation achievement has been the dispersion of evidence-based effective behavioral interventions (DEBIs) for essential and auxiliary HIV avoidance among people, little gatherings, and communities. These mediations help to guarantee that those people at the most serious risk for HIV transmission or acquisition can get escalated backing to reduce the chance practices and receive defensive procedures for their well-being and the health of their partners.

Remaining Challenges

Regardless of these successes, a few difficulties remain. HIV/AIDS keeps on being the main source of illness and death in the United States. An expected 252,000 – 312,000 HIV-contaminated people in the United States are unconscious of their HIV disease. Not exclusively are those at high risk for transmitting HIV to other people, and yet they are considerably less likely to take advantage of effective medical treatments.

Certain subpopulations stay at expanded risk. MSM represents roughly 45% of recently reported HIV/AIDS cases and almost 54% of total AIDS analysis. An ongoing review showed that in a few enormous U.S. urban communities, roughly one out of four MSM reviewed in social venues is infected with HIV, and almost half of

MSM are unaware of their HIV diseases. Besides, youthful MSM was most drastically averse to realize they were infected, and MSM from racial/ethnic minority populations reliably showed higher prevalence than white MSM. The yearly HIV rate among MSM is high, going from 1.2% to 8.0%. Racial and ethnic minority communities also are disproportionately influenced by HIV/AIDS.

During 2001 – 2004, in 35 zones with HIV revealing, 51% of all new HIV/AIDS analysis were among blacks, who represent around 13% of the U.S. populace. Of these, 11% (12,650) of HIV/AIDS diagnoses in men were dark men who were infected through hetero contact, and 54% (23,820) of HIV/AIDS cases in ladies were in dark ladies infected through heterosexual contact. Today, ladies represent roughly one-fourth of all new HIV/AIDS cases, and in 2002, HIV disease was the main source of death for dark matured ladies of 25-34 years.

A scaling up of the diffusion of effective behavioral interventions (e.g., DEBIs) is required; however, limitations exist in CDC's capacity to meet current preparing and specialized help needs, just as states' capacities to actualize them generally. Different holes incorporate the absence of information concerning the adequacy of adjusting DEBIs to all in at-risk populations.

In numerous districts, the network level workforce may be debilitated by wearing down, weariness, and inadequate program skills. Changing the open impression of HIV/AIDS in the United States, combined with the across the board availability of highly active antiretroviral treatment, has led to the widespread belief that AIDS is never again an issue or a serious disease in the United States. Although 26% of people in the United States consider AIDS as a top health concern for the country (second just to malignant growth [35%]), those who consider it to be the main medical issue has declined during the previous years. Complacency, stigma, and discrimination persist, and all decrease inspiration among people and networks to receive risk decrease practices, get tested for HIV, and access anticipation and treatment services.

New Strategies

Regardless of these difficulties, generous open doors stay to improve and show the viability of HIV-prevention measures. New strategies should be joined with a scaling up of customarily successful mediations that are custom-made for the local study of disease transmission and setting to increase public health impact despite resource constraints.

Partnerships: Eliminating HIV/AIDS in the United States can't be achieved by any single office or gathering. It will require general health organizations containing people, communities, agencies, and the private sector. Strong partnerships are particularly crucial to address disgrace and separation and to advance more prominent acknowledgment of those living with HIV/AIDS. Strict and business networks and remedial and emotional health services all should be a piece of a national mobilization in the prevention of HIV transmission. An improved, coordinated effort across government organizations is additionally required to give a bound together public health infrastructure devoted to examining, anticipation, treatment, care, and rehabilitative services for people influenced by HIV/AIDS.

Expanded access to voluntary HIV testing: For the assessment of a million people living with HIV who are unaware of their HIV disease, testing is the entryway to lifesaving treatment. People who realize they are infected with HIV are bound to find a way to keep themselves from transmitting the infection to other people. To decrease the number of people with undiagnosed HIV infections, continued development of access to and take-up of HIV testing will be required. This decrease can be achieved by making willful HIV testing a standard piece of clinical consideration, reducing the boundaries to HIV testing, and guaranteeing simple access to new fast HIV tests that, in numerous purviews, can be performed via trained people who are not clinicians.

Prevention messages focused on both HIV-positive and HIV-negative people. Giving socially and relevantly fitting messages is fundamental to help people at risk avoid contracting HIV disease and helping the individuals who are infected with HIV abstain from transmitting the infection. Anticipation messages also need to focus on the job of liquor and medication maltreatment in HIV. Substance abuse (using infusion medications, liquor, or methamphetamines) can encourage risky behaviors among persons who may find some way or another to shield themselves as well as other people from HIV. Preventing substance misuse and expanding access to substance-misuse treatment are instances of successful mediations for decreasing HIV transmission.

They have integrated prevention programs. Government, state, and nearby counteraction measures are more focused on maximizing public health sway for some random program. One way to deal with expanding program adequacy is by expanding the improvement and implementation of incorporated HIV-anticipation programs. A few coordinated projects exist the country over, consolidating HIV, sexually transmitted disease (STD), viral hepatitis, psychological health, and substance misuse services. Successful integration requires that program chiefs:

1) Better characterize program joining objectives.
2) Recognize best practices in the field and guarantee that they are spread and implemented widely.
3) Implement policies and regulations that upgrade and bolster incorporation at nearby levels.
4) Assess the most cost-effective strategies.

Improved observation of new HIV infections. Dependable, populace based information is fundamental to follow the HIV epidemic, and target prevention quantifies precisely. For quite a long time, AIDS surveillance has been a foundation of national, state, and local efforts to monitor the degree and effect of the HIV pandemic. However, AIDS observation information never again precisely describes the full level of the pestilence because successful treatments have eased back the movement of the disease. Since 1999, CDC has suggested that states direct HIV detailing, utilizing a similar name-based methodology presently utilized for AIDS observation across the nation. Right now, 43 states and five regions utilize private, name-based HIV case reporting. A few of the rest of the states expect to actualize name-based HIV observation in 2006. Also, in 2006, information from another national HIV incidence surveillance system will give the most exact appraisals of new HIV contaminations. This information joined with improved surveillance of the examples and circulations of risk behaviors in the population will refine the focus on and delivery of HIV-prevention efforts.

New prevention technologies: Certain avoidance advancements still being worked on, including pre-exposure prophylaxis, microbicides, and immunizations, are probably not going to give full assurance against HIV and may offer practically zero insurance against different STDs like gonorrhea and Chlamydia infections. Also, they won't prevent unwanted pregnancies. Rather, innovations are bound to be fused into the range of devices for extensive ways to deal with disease prevention. Effective behavior-change projects will even now be expected to address conceivable social freedom (i.e., proceeding or coming back to high-chance practices when one feels assured) among people who get these interventions. Prevention counseling that addresses to educated decision and consent. The HIV-prevention practices of abstinence and delay of sexual debut, being monogamous, having fewer sex partners, and utilizing condoms accurately and reliably, as well as other reproductive health needs (e.g., STD treatment and family arranging), must be fused with these new prevention interventions.

Special Issue of MMWR

HIV/AIDS remains a potentially deadly chronic disease. Prevention of HIV infection requires taking responsibility from people at risk, people infected, and society in general. Prevention efforts need to keep pace with an evolving epidemic. Above all, younger ages, who probably won't recall the deadlier beginning of the scourge, consistently need to get essential HIV-prevention messages. A quarter-century after the first provision of details regarding AIDS, MMWR devotes this issue to reviews on the pestilence, including changing the study of disease transmission of HIV/AIDS, the public health achievement in reducing perinatal transmission of HIV, and the advancement of measures to prevent HIV/AIDS.

The Development of Research, Treatment, and Prevention

Azidothymidine, otherwise called *zidovudine*, was presented in 1987 as the main treatment for HIV. Researchers additionally created medications to decrease mother-to-child transmission.

In 1997, exceptionally active antiretroviral treatment (HAART) turned into the new treatment standard. It caused a 47 percent decrease in death rates.

The Food and Drug Administration (FDA) approved the main fast HIV diagnostic test pack in November 2002. The test unit allowed emergency clinics to give results with 99.6 percent accuracy in 20 minutes.

Also, in 2003, the CDC detailed that 40,000 new infections happened every year. The greater part of those transmissions originated from individuals who didn't realize they were infected. It was later found the number was more like 56,300 diseases. This number generally remains the equivalent since the late 1990s.

The World Health Organization set an objective to carry treatment to 3 million individuals by 2005. By 2010, about 5.25 million individuals had treatment, and 1.2 million individuals would begin treatment.

Current Treatment

The FDA endorsed Combivir in 1997. Combivir joins two medications into a single medication, making HIV meds simpler to take.

Scientists kept on making new plans and mixes to improve treatment results. By 2010, there were up to 20 diverse treatment options and non-exclusive medications, which helped lower costs. The FDA keeps on affirming HIV clinical items, regulating:

- Product approval
- Warnings
- Safety guidelines
- Label updates

Starting in 2017, Trusted Source has shown that an individual living with HIV on standard antiretroviral treatment that decreases the infection to undetectable levels in the blood can't transmit HIV to a partner during sex. The present accord among clinical experts is that "undetectable = un-transmittable."

The Social Reaction to HIV

Stigma in the Early Years

When initially scarcely any instances of AIDS developed, people believed the disease was just shrunk by men who had sex with men. The CDC called this infection GRIDS, or gay-related immunodeficiency syndrome. Not long after, the CDC distributed a case definition calling the disease AIDS.

The public response was negative in the early stretches of the pestilence. In 1983, a New York specialist was undermined with eviction, leading to the main AIDS discrimination lawsuit.

Bathhouses all over the nation shut because of high-chance sexual action. A few schools likewise banned youngsters with HIV from joining in.

In 1987, the United States set a movement prohibition on guests and settlers with HIV. President Obama lifted this boycott in 2010.

The United States government opposed financing needle exchange programs (NEPs) because of the war on drugs. NEPs were demonstrated to be viable at decreasing HIV transmission. Some accept that this opposition represents 4,400 to 9,700 avoidable diseases.

Government Support

Consistently, the government keeps on subsidizing HIV- and AIDS-related:

- Systems of care
- Counseling
- Testing services
- Treatment
- Studies and research

In 1985, President Ronald Reagan called research about AIDS "a top need" for his organization. President Clinton facilitated the main White House Conference on HIV and AIDS and required a vaccine to look into focus. This center later opened in 1999.

Mainstream Society Opens Up Discussions About HIV

Entertainer Rock Hudson was the primary significant public figure to recognize he had AIDS. After he died in 1985, he left $250,000 to set up an AIDS establishment. Elizabeth Taylor was the national director until she died in 2011. Princess Diana also stood out as truly newsworthy after she warmly greeted somebody with HIV.

Mainstream society symbol Freddie Mercury, the artist for the band Queen, additionally died from AIDS-related sicknesses in 1991. From that point forward, numerous different big names have revealed that they're HIV-positive. All the more as of late, Charlie Sheen reported his status on national TV.

In 1995, the National Association of People with AIDS established National HIV Testing Day. Associations, shows, and communities keep on battling the marks of disgrace connected to this disease.

Following the Legislative Issues of Blood Bans

Before the epidemic, U.S. blood donation centers didn't screen for HIV. When they began doing as such in 1985, men who engaged in sexual relations with men were restricted from giving blood. On December 2015, the FDA lifted a portion of its limitations. The current strategy says that givers can give blood if they have not had sexual contact with another man for at any rate one year.

Ongoing Medication Advancement for HIV Prevention

In July 2012, the FDA approved pre-exposure prophylaxis (PrEP). PrEP is a drug that appeared to bring down the risk of contracting HIV from sexual activity or needle use. The treatment requires taking the prescription every day.

Doctors prescribe PrEP for individuals who are involved with somebody who has HIV. The US Preventive Services Task Force prescribes it for all individuals at an increased risk of HIV.

Individuals who may profit from PrEP include:

• People in a non-monogamous relationship with a partner who is HIV-negative (PrEP lessens the risk of transmitting HIV to a partner)

• People who have had butt-centric sex without a condom or who have gotten a sexually transmitted disease (STD) in the previous half year

• People who have sex with people

• People who have infused drugs, or have been in medicated treatment, or shared needles in the previous a half year

- People who routinely have different sexual partners of obscure HIV status, particularly if they infuse drugs

PrEP appeared to decrease the hazard for HIV infection by more than 90 percent.

What Impact Does HIV Have on the Body?

HIV attacks a particular sort of resistant framework cell in the body. It's known as the CD4 assistant cell or T cell. At the point when HIV destroys this cell, it becomes harder for the body to ward off different infections.

At the point when HIV is left untreated, even a minor disease, for example, a virus can be substantially more extreme. This is because the body experiences issues reacting to new diseases.

In addition to the fact that HIV attacks CD4 cells, it also utilizes the cells to increase the infection. HIV attacks CD4 cells by utilizing their replication apparatus to make new duplicates of the infection. This, at last, makes the CD4 cells swell and burst.

When the virus has destroyed a specific number of CD4 cells, and the CD4 count drops under 200, an individual will have progressed to AIDS.

But, note that headways in HIV treatment have made it workable for some individuals with HIV to live more, healthier lives.

How Is HIV Transmitted?

HIV is transmitted through contact with the following organic liquids, from 'well on the way' to prompt HIV transmission to least likely:

- Blood

- Semen

- Vaginal liquid

- Breast milk

Sex without a condom and sharing needles, even tattoo or piercing needles, can transmit HIV. However, if an HIV-positive individual can achieve viral suppression, at that point, they'll not be able to transmit HIV to others through sexual contact.

As indicated by the Centers for Disease Control and Prevention (CDC) Trusted Source, an individual has arrived at viral suppression when they have less than 200 duplicates of HIV RNA per milliliter of blood.

What Are the Phases of HIV?

HIV Is Characterized by 3 Phases: Acute HIV, Chronic HIV, and AIDS

HIV doesn't, in every case, increase quickly. Whenever left untreated, it can take a very long time for an individual's resistant framework to be influenced enough to give indications of immune dysfunction and different diseases. View a course of events of HIV symptoms.

Indeed, even without indications, HIV can, in any case, be available in the body and can be transmitted. Getting satisfactory treatment that results in viral suppression stops the movement of safe brokenness and AIDS. Satisfactory treatment additionally helps a damaged immune system to recover.

When an individual contracts HIV, the acute infection takes place immediately.

Side effects of the acute disease may happen days to weeks after the infection has been contacted. During this time, the infection is multiplying quickly in the body, unchecked.

This underlying HIV stage can bring about influenza-like indications. Instances of these side effects include:

- Fever

- Headache

- Rash

- Swollen lymph hubs

- Fatigue

- Myalgias, or muscle pain

However, not all individuals with HIV experience initial influenza-like side effects.

This season's flu virus side effects result from the increase in the multiplication of HIV and far-reaching disease in the body. During this time, the measure of CD4 cells begins to fall rapidly. The resistant framework at that point kicks in, causing CD4 levels to rise by and by. But, the CD4 levels may not come back to their pre-HIV height.

In addition to potentially causing symptoms, the acute stage is where individuals with HIV have the best possibility of transmitting the infection to other people. This is because HIV levels are high right now. The acute stage regularly keeps going between a little while and months.

How Does Chronic HIV Influence the Body?

The chronic HIV stage is known as the idle or asymptomatic stage. During this stage, an individual typically won't have the same number of side effects as they did during the intense stage. This is because the infection doesn't multiply as quickly.

However, a person can, in any case, transmit HIV if the infection is left untreated, and they keep on having a detectable viral load. Without treatment, the interminable HIV stage can keep going for a long time before progressing to AIDS.

Advances in antiretroviral medicines have altogether improved the viewpoint for individuals living with HIV. With appropriate treatment, numerous individuals who are HIV-positive can achieve viral suppression and live long, solid lives. Become familiar with HIV and the future.

CHAPTER 10 - SERIOUS ACUTE RESPIRATORY SYNDROME (SARS)

Serious acute respiratory syndrome (SARS) is a viral respiratory illness brought about by a coronavirus, called SARS-related coronavirus (SARS-CoV). SARS was first announced in Asia in February 2003. The disease spread to more than two dozen countries in North America, South America, Europe, and Asia before the SARS worldwide episode of 2003 was contained.

As of now, there is no known SARS transmission anywhere in the world. The latest human SARS-CoV disease cases were accounted for in China in April 2004 out of an episode coming about because of laboratory-acquired infections. CDC and its partners, including the World Health Organization, keep on checking the SARS circumstance globally.

In November 2002, a type of atypical pneumonia called severe acute respiratory syndrome (SARS) started spreading quickly around the globe, provoking the World Health Organization (WHO) to declare the disease "an overall wellbeing danger." At the focal point of the outbreak was China, where the SARS outbreak infected more than 5,300 individuals and killed 349 across the country. History is loaded with ironies: the epidemic got China, from the start, unprepared to defeat the disease 45 years after Mao Zedong bade "Goodbye to the God of Plagues."

The SARS epidemic was not just a public medical issue. Surely, it caused the most extreme socio-political emergency for the Chinese service since the 1989 Tiananmen crackdown. The outbreak of the disease fueled fears among market analysts that China's economy was set out toward a serious downturn. A lethal time of hesitation concerning data sharing and activity produced tension, panic, and rumor-mongering all over the nation and undermined the government's efforts to make a milder picture of itself in the worldwide field. As Premier Wen Jiabao called attention to it in a cabinet meeting on the pandemic, "the well-being and security of the individuals, by and large, is a condition of change, advancement, and strength; and China's national interest and global picture are in question. In the weeks that followed, the Chinese government launched a campaign against SARS, viably bringing the infection under control in late June and eliminating all known cases by mid-August.

While it was a test for China's public health infrastructure, the course of the plague also brought up significant issues about the limit and elements of the Chinese political structure and its capacity to address future outbreaks. What represented the underlying government choices to retain data from general society and make a little movement against the sickness, and then the resulting emotional move in government approach toward SARS? For what reason was the service ready to contain the spread of SARS in a moderately brief period? What exercises have the legislature drawn from the emergency? A political investigation of the emergency isn't just showing essential linkages between China's political framework and its example of crisis management.

Additionally, it reveals insight into the government's capacity to deal with the following ailment episode. While issues in the formal institutional structure and bureaucratic limit represented the initial denial and inaction, the institutional powers released from the landscape of state-society relations prompted sensational changes in the structure and content of the government approach toward SARS. Through mass mobilization, the government successfully brought the disease under control. While these improvements are empowering,

China's ability to successfully prevent and contain future infectious disease outbreaks stays questionable. Prevention and control programs are as yet disturbed by issues in motivation setting, strategy making, and usage, which, thus, can be attributed to its political framework. A more advantageous China in this manner requests some essential changes in the political system.

The Making of a Crisis

Looking back, China's health system appeared to be at first to react moderately well to the disease's development. The soonest instance of SARS is thought to have happened in Foshan, a city southwest of Guangzhou in the Guangdong area, in mid-November 2002. It was later also found in Heyuan and Zhongshan in Guangdong. This "strange disease" alerted Chinese health personnel as right on time as mid-December. On January 2, a team of health experts was sent to Heyuan and analyzed the disease as an infection brought about by a specific infection. A Chinese doctor, who was accountable for treating a patient from Heyuan in a medical clinic in Guangzhou, immediately revealed the disease to a local anti-epidemic station. We have the motivation to accept that the local hostile to pandemic station alarmed the common health authority about the infection. This results in the agency reporting to the provincial government and the Ministry of Health a while later, since the main group of specialists sent by the Ministry showed up at Guangzhou on January 20, and the new provincial government (who took over on January 20) requested an examination of the sickness almost at the same time. A combined health specialists from the Ministry and the area were dispatched to Zhongshan and finished an examination report on the unknown disease.

On January 27, the report was sent to the provincial health department and, apparently, to the Ministry of Health in Beijing. The report was marked "top secret," which meant that only top provincial health officials could open it.

Further government response to the developing disease, in any case, was postponed by the issues of data stream inside the Chinese progressive system. For 3 days, there were no authorized provincial health officials available to open the document. After the report was finally read, the provincial department delivered a notice to emergency clinics over the province. However, few health workers were alerted by the notice because most were in the midst of a get-away for the Chinese New Year. Meanwhile, the general population was kept uninformed about the disease. As indicated by the Implementing Regulations on the State Secrets Law concerning the treatment of public health-related data, any event of infectious diseases ought to be named a state mystery before they are "declared by the Ministry of Health or organs approved by the Ministry." As it were, until the Ministry decided to make data about the blackout public, any physician or journalist who wrote about the disease would risk being persecuted for leaking state secrets.

A virtual news power outage about SARS, therefore, proceeded well into February.

The initial failure to advise general society increased tensions, fear, and far-reaching theory. On February 8, reports about a "deadly flu" started to be sent through short messages on cell phones in Guangzhou. At night, words like bird influenza and *Bacillus anthracis* began to show up on some local Internet sites. On February 10, the news showed up in the nearby media that recognized the presence of the infection and recorded some preventive measures, including improving ventilation, utilizing vinegar fumes to sterilize the air, and washing hands now and again. Reacting to the advice, residents in Guangzhou and different urban areas cleared pharmacy shelves of antibiotics and flu medication. In certain urban communities, even the vinegar was sold out. The panic spread rapidly in Guangdong and was felt even in different areas.

On February 11, Guangdong health authorities, at last, ended the quietness by holding question and answer sessions about the infection. The common wellbeing authorities detained a total of 305 atypical pneumonia cases in the area. The authorities additionally conceded that there were no compelling medications to treat the disease and that the outbreak was just probably contained. From that point on, data about the disease was accounted for to the general population through the news media. However, meanwhile, they play down the risk of the disease. Guangzhou regional government on February 11 went so far as to declare the disease seemed to be "comprehensively" under successful control. Accordingly, while the panic was incidentally relieved, the openness additionally lost vigilance about the infection. When a few reports started to question the government's treatment of the outbreak, the common purposeful publicity department again stopped giving an account of the disease on February 23. This news power outage was kept during the approach the National People's Congress in March, and government specialists shared little data to the World Health Organization until early April.

What Is the Cause of SARS?

The SARS infection spreads by close person-to-person contact. Transmission likely happens by beads created when an infected person sneezes or coughs. Bead spread can happen when airborne beads, delivered by a cough and sneeze, are saved on the mucous membranes of the mouth, nose, or eyes of an individual up to 3 feet away. The infection can also be spread when an individual touches a surface contaminated with the droplets, as was found on numerous medical clinic surfaces, including lift catches. Oral-fecal transmission of SARS may likewise happen. Unprotected medical services workers were a significant risk of getting the infection during the outbreaks.

SARS infection duplicates in both the lungs and gastrointestinal tract tissues. But, tissue tests show the greatest harm that occurs in the lung alveoli (air sacs) where lung work is undermined, creating a serious breathing issue regularly named acute respiratory distress syndrome (ARDS).

What Are SARS Risk Factors?

SARS risk factors incorporate an introduction to somebody infected with the infection or people going in an area where an outbreak of SARS is happening. Other risk factors incorporate, for example, diabetes and chronic hepatitis B. Human services laborers who were presented to SARS patients in the past episodes are additionally at expanded risk of contracting the disease.

What Are the Signs and Symptoms of SARS?

Side effects of SARS can be like those of other viral diseases. The principal symptoms start two to seven days after the introduction and incorporate at least one of the following:

- Fever (temperature of more than 100.4 F)

- Headache

- Fatigue (tiredness)

- Muscle aches and pain

- Malaise (a feeling of general discomfort)

- Decreased craving

- Diarrhea

Respiratory indications are created at least three days after the presentation. Respiratory indications incorporate one of a greater amount of the following:

• Dry hack

• Shortness of breath

• Runny nose and sore throat (phenomenal)

By day seven to 10 of the disease, practically all patients with research center proof of SARS infection have pneumonia that could be recognized in the lungs on X-ray films. Respiratory pain happens in certain patients. This side effect is a worry for the patient and the specialists since it proposes the sickness is becoming more severe.

When Should Someone Seek Medical Care for Possible Exposure to SARS?

Obtaining SARS infection is generally connected with movement to a nation where SARS has been accounted for or contact with an ill individual who has quite recently come back from that country. Individuals who might have been presented to SARS or SARS-like flare-ups, later on, should look for clinical care promptly and are encouraged to call a specialist if a fever or respiratory symptoms occur and tell healthcare workers that conceivable presentation to SARS may have happened.

What Specialists Treat SARS?

Primary-care physicians may treat the symptoms of mellow SARS infections in certain patients. Moderate to extreme SARS-infected patients may require infectious-disease, basic consideration, pulmonologists, and hospitalists as masters to help care for these patients. In the U.S., CDC masters ought to be educated immediately if an outbreak of SARS or SARS-like disease happens.

What Tests Do Physicians Use to Diagnose SARS?

Beginning tests for individuals thought to have SARS incorporate the following:

• Chest X-ray films

• Pulse oximetry (a test wherein a test associated with a PC is set on the finger or ear to gauge oxygen saturation in the blood).

• Blood profiles

- Sputum (fluid from the respiratory tract) Gram stain and culture

- If SARS infection disease is suspected, the CDC ought to be informed; the CDC has particular tests (RT-PCR and EIA) to identify the infection. These tests are not normally available to most labs, although some state labs may have availability.

- Testing for viral specialists, for example, flu A, flu B, fledgling influenza, West Nile infection, *Bacillus anthracis*, and respiratory syncytial virus (RSV) might be done to preclude these issues or diseases that might be mistaken for SARS. Particularly if there is no initial suspicion that SARS brings about the issue and if SARS testing isn't readily available.

- Urinary antigen testing for Legionella and pneumococcal species (two reasons for bacterial pneumonia)

Are There Home Remedies for SARS?

Follow the rules depicted in Prevention to constrain the spread and transmission of SARS disease. Patients are typically treated in an emergency clinic in case they are confirmed to have SARS.

What Are SARS Treatments?

By now, no particular treatment exists for SARS, although different medicines have been tried with indistinct achievement. Authorities on infectious diseases and pneumonic consideration and others ought to be engaged with the consideration of SARS patients. Clinical medicines that have been tried include corticosteroids, antiviral specialists, interferon, and different antibody preparations, nitric oxide, and a customary Chinese prescription named *glycyrrhizin* (a compound found in licorice roots). A large portion of these medications has not been focused enough to prove effectiveness. Most hospitalized patients require steady consideration, for example, supplemental oxygen or mechanical ventilation.

People with confirmed or suspected SARS ought to be isolated and given aggressive treatment in a medical clinic. Mechanical ventilation (a device that aids an individual's breathing) and basic consideration might be vital due to respiratory distress.

What Medications Treat SARS?

In a portion of the main instances of SARS, antibiotics were utilized with no achievement. When it was resolved that SARS was an infection, the antiviral medication ribavirin was utilized, some of the time in combination with corticosteroids. But, data is constrained on whether these medications will decrease the general disease severity and death from SARS.

How Often Is Follow-up Needed After SARS Treatment?

SARS was (and potentially might be again later on) a serious viral illness that requires brief clinical attention and hospitalization. When the individual is released from the medical clinic, line up care with a doctor should be scheduled.

By What Means Can People Prevent SARS?

Individuals in direct or close contact with somebody who has had SARS were at the most serious risk for the disease. Individuals with SARS or those at risk for SARS ought to follow the guidelines outlined below. The WHO and CDC have set up rules to help in the prevention and spread of SARS.

• Limit time outside of the home. Individuals with SARS ought not to go to work, school, kid care offices, or any open spot until 10 days after their fever has finished and their respiratory symptoms are improving.

• Wash hands as often as possible with cleanser and heated water, utilize a liquor based hand rub, or both, particularly in the wake of being in contact with organic liquids, for example, respiratory fluids or urine.

• Wear dispensable gloves when in contact with organic liquids from an individual with SARS. After use, discard the gloves quickly and altogether wash the hands.

• Wear a surgical mask.

• Cover the nose and mouth with a tissue when sneezing or coughing.

• Do not share eating utensils, towels, or bedding. Completely wash these things with cleanser and high temp water after use by an infected individual.

• Use a household disinfectant on any surface that might be infected; for example, ledges or door handles. Wear dispensable gloves while cleaning these surfaces.

• Follow these rules for at any rate 10 days after the side effects have settled.

What Is the Prognosis for SARS?

SARS can bring about serious illness and medical complications that require hospitalization, intensive care treatment, and mechanical ventilation. The latest numbers show that the death rate from SARS is higher than that of flu or other basic respiratory tract infections. Complications incorporate adjusted lung work, polyneuropathy, and avascular necrosis.

The general passing (death) rate from SARS is about 10%. Age is a hazard factor and assumes an enormous job in the guess. Patients under 24 years old have a death rate of about 1%, while those more than 65 years old can have a half or higher death rate. Other risk factors incorporate patients with chronic hepatitis B infection, hepatitis from any reason, diabetes, *lymphopenia*, *leukocytosis*, and high cytokine levels early (first week) in the SARS disease. 2009 H1N1 Pandemic (H1N1pdm09 infection).

In the spring of 2009, the novel flu A (H1N1) virus emerged. It was detected first in the United States and spread rapidly over the United States and the world. This new H1N1 infection contained a one of a kind blend of flu qualities not recently identified in animals or people. This infection was assigned as flu A (H1N1) pdm09 infection.

After ten years, work keeps on improving on flu, prevent sickness, and getting ready for the following pandemic.

The 2009 H1N1 Pandemic: A New Flu Virus Emerges

The (H1N1) pdm09 infection was altogether different from H1N1 infections that were coursing at the hour of the pandemic. Few young people had any current immunity (as distinguished by counteracting agent reaction) to the (H1N1) pdm09 infection. Yet, almost 33% of individuals more than 60 years of age had antibodies against this infection, likely from presentation to a more seasoned H1N1 infection before in their lives. Since the (H1N1) pdm09 infection was altogether different from flowing H1N1 infections, vaccination with seasonal flu vaccines offered minimal cross-security against (H1N1) pdm09 infection disease. While a monovalent (H1N1) pdm09 antibody was created, it was not available in enormous amounts until late November—after the pinnacle of disease, when the subsequent wave had traveled every way in the United States. From April 12, 2009 to April 10, 2010, CDC evaluated there were 60.8 million cases (run: 43.3-89.3 million), 274,304 hospitalizations (run:

195,086-402,719), and 12,469 deaths (run: 8868-18,306) in the United States due to the (H1N1) pdm09 infection.

Furthermore, CDC evaluated that 151,700-575,400 people worldwide died from (H1N1) pdm09 virus infection during the primary year the infection circulated. Globally, 80 percent of (H1N1) pdm09 infection-related deaths were assessed to have happened in individuals more youthful than 65 years old. This contrasts extraordinarily from the run of the mill regular flu pestilences, during which around 70 percent to 90 percent of deaths are evaluated to happen in individuals 65 years and more seasoned.

Although the 2009 influenza pandemic influenced kids and young and middle-aged adults, the effect of the (H1N1) pdm09 infection on the worldwide population during the primary year was less extreme than that of past pandemics. Evaluations of pandemic flu mortality extended from 0.03 percent of the total population during the 1968 H3N2 pandemic to 1 percent to 3 percent of the total population during the 1918 H1N1 pandemic. It is evaluated that 0.001 percent to 0.007 percent of the total population died of respiratory complications related to (H1N1) pdm09 virus infection during the initial year the virus circulated.

The United States mounted a complex, multi-faceted, and long-term response to the pandemic, as summarized in The 2009 H1N1 Pandemic: Summary Highlights, April 2009-April 2010. On August 10, 2010, WHO pronounced a conclusion to the worldwide 2009 H1N1 flu pandemic. However, (H1N1) pdm09 virus continues circling as an occasional influenza infection and consistently causes illness, hospitalization, and deaths worldwide.

CHAPTER 11 - EBOLA

The Ebola virus disease — earlier known as Ebola hemorrhagic fever — is a rare and often dangerous malady in people brought about by infection with one of four Ebola infection strains — Zaire, Sudan, Bundibugyo, or Tai Forest.

What Are the Side Effects of Ebola?

Manifestations of Ebola incorporate high body temperatures, headache, abdominal pain, diarrhea, vomiting, and internal and external bleeding, such as gums and stool. It very well may be hard to separate Ebola from different illnesses, for example, intestinal sickness, typhoid fever, and meningitis. Side effects can show up from two to 21 days after getting the disease. Individuals who have gotten the sickness can't offer it to others until side effects show up.

Is Ebola Treatable?

There is no proven, licensed treatment for the virus, yet treating early indications and rehydration with IV liquids improve survival rates.

Potential medicines, including blood, immunological, and tranquilize treatments, are being created, and a trial Ebola vaccine proved highly powerful in a 2015 trial in Guinea.

The Ebola antibody is being utilized in the Democratic Republic of Congo to offer insusceptibility to individuals' at the most elevated risk for the sickness, including groups of individuals who are infected. The vaccine proved safe and effective before testing; however, it isn't yet authorized across the board use.

How Is Ebola Spread?

Ebola is extremely infectious, which means direct contact with a limited quantity of the infection can lead to infection. However, it doesn't spread through the air. Individuals become infected with the virus by close contact with infected animals, once in a while by butchering and eating shrubbery meat, or by presentation to the organic liquids of infected individuals. Sexual contact additionally spreads the virus.

The bodies of the individuals who have passed on from Ebola carry high concentrations of the infection that can spread to others through contact. Giving safe and dignified burials to individuals is critical to forestall the spread of the disease.

For What Reason Did the 2014 Outbreak in West Africa Spread So Quickly?

The Ebola virus was relatively unknown in West Africa, so it infected and killed individuals for quite a long time before being identified. It was the principal Ebola episode to spread unchecked through urban areas; the capital urban areas of Guinea, Sierra Leone, and Liberia. The flare-up was followed back to a 2-year-old child infected in Guinea in December 2013, a quarter of a year before the outbreak was declared.

The infection spread quickly where infected individuals were brought back home or died at home, and their bodies were washed and arranged for burial by family members, as indicated by tradition.

For What Reason Was Ebola So Difficult to Stop?

Medical services in West Africa weren't all generally well staffed or prepared to deal with the disease. Without early diagnosis and notification, the global clinical community was delayed in giving assets to control the spread of the outbreak.

The impacts of the epidemic were most exceedingly terrible in Sierra Leone as far as the all-out quantities of cases and the quantities of cases per capita are concerned. The country's health system was delicate and short of human services workers, weaknesses dating from the common war that finished 10 years prior.

Is There a Risk of an Ebola Episode in the United States?

The U.S. Communities for Disease Control and Prevention says Ebola is extremely unlikely to happen in the U.S. since the disease isn't spread by casual contact. There have been a couple of cases occurring in the U.S. among individuals who have traveled where the disease is found, and that could happen once more.

Similar strategies used to control outbreaks of the disease would be effective in preventing its spread in the U.S. These include identifying and isolating cases, following potential contacts, thinking about patients in uncommonly planned Ebola treatment focuses, and guaranteeing protected and dignified burials.

How might I help survivors of Ebola?

• Pray for the survivors: Dear Lord, you mended bodies, minds, and spirits during your service. We request that your healing power be shown to the young ladies and young men, ladies, and men whose lives were compromised by the episode of Ebola in West Africa. May they know the comfort and assurance of your quality? May the individuals, who grieve the loss of loved ones, find their hope in you?

• Sponsor a youngster in Sierra Leone as an individual method to demonstrate God's love to a child in need.

World Vision's Reaction to the Ebola Outbreak

At the time Ebola struck Sierra Leone, World Vision was at that point working in 25 region improvement programs benefiting around 58,000 kids and their families. Our first concern was for their health. We immediately acknowledged that we would need to step out in confidence past our typical improvement work to make a strong contribution to the completion of the epidemic.

Expanding on 20 years of grassroots association in Sierra Leone, we got together with communities, partner agencies, and each level of government in the fight against Ebola. There were no deaths among the World Vision-supported children and their families.

A 2016 investigation of World Vision's reaction by Johns Hopkins University showed that the organization is a trusted source of Ebola anticipation data, and World Vision's religious methodology is successful in affecting individuals to change risky behavior and look for medical attention.

During the crisis response, World Vision contacted 1.6 million individuals through these and different activities:

Health and Safety
- World Vision assembled globally to convey 5.4 million individual defensive gear things, including suits, gloves, face covers, and goggles to use in Sierra Leone medical clinics and health centers and gave cleanliness units to schools. Long-term World Vision partner McKesson, the biggest social insurance services organization in the U.S., gave 200 pallets of medical relief supplies, enough to address Sierra Leone's issues for five months.

Awareness and Prevention
- World Vision-prepared staff organized massive awareness, prevention, and instruction battles to

shield kids from the disease through radio and house-to-house data sharing.

- Staff prepared more than 2,000 influential local leaders, including Christian and Muslim ministers, conventional confidence healers, and cutting edge community health workers to deliver messages on Ebola awareness and prevention. "When such a significant number of networks face such terrible suffering, the congregation must be there to combat fear, stigma, isolation, and hopelessness with both love and substantial help," said Bruno Col, World Vision communications chief in West Africa.

Safe and Dignified Burials

- World Vision handled 800 trained burial teams, with two other guide organizations, that performed 29,201 burials to prevent transmission of the disease, while families concerned have to grieve and protect tradition.
- World Vision and its humanitarian partners, alongside the burial workers, like 53-year-old Ebola survivor Maseray Kamara, were granted the Bond International Humanitarian Award. The award recognized the mental fortitude and caring of those on the bleeding edges of Ebola avoidance during the outbreak. "This acknowledgment is huge support

after all the suffering we have found in Sierra Leone and across West Africa," says Grace Kargbo, a World Vision Sierra Leone internment group director. "These fearless spirits have gotten little acknowledgment at home and abroad. They have regularly been shunned, ostracized, denounced because they are burial workers."

Follow an Ebola burial group giving a safe and dignified burial for Betty Thomas, 42, from the Moyamba locale of Sierra Leone. While showing up at her home, the group put on the defensive gear, a 10-to 15-minute procedure that entailed every one putting on three sets of gloves and wrapping and removing her body while showering disinfectant. A minister at that point drove short assistance, including the Lord's Prayer, and Betty's body was removed to be covered. Her family members followed the group to her grave.

Social and Economic Recovery

- World Vision helped families and communities recover and assemble strength with reserve funds bunches for financial recovery, cultivating upgrades, and backing for reintegrating Ebola vagrants and survivors into family and community life. We prepared teachers to give psychosocial backing to youngsters coming back to schools as well as organized and repaid volunteers to get ready schools to reopen.

CHAPTER 12 - PANDEMIC RISK FACTORS

Pandemic risk, as noted, is driven by the joined impacts of spark risk and spread risk. The foci of both risk factors frequently cover, particularly in some LMICs, (for example, in Central and West Africa and Southeast Asia), making these areas especially vulnerable against pandemics and their negative results.

Spark Risk

A zoonotic spark could emerge from the presentation of a pathogen from either domesticated animals or wildlife. Zoonoses from domesticated animals are packed in regions with thick livestock domesticated production systems, including zones of China, India, Japan, the United States, and Western Europe. Key drivers for spark risk from domesticated animals incorporate concentrated and broad cultivating and domesticated animals' production systems and live creature markets, just as the potential for contact among animals and wildlife reservoirs. Natural life zoonosis hazard is appropriated unquestionably more broadly, with foci in China, India,

West and Central Africa, and the Amazon Basin. Risk drivers incorporate social components (for example, bush meat chasing and utilization of animal-based traditional medicines), common asset extraction, (for example, sylviculture and logging), the extension of streets into natural life living spaces, and ecological elements (counting the degree and dispersion of animal diversity).

Spread Risk

After a spark or importation, the risk that a pathogen will spread inside a population is affected by pathogen-specific factors (including genetic adaptation and method of transmission) and human population-level factors. For example, the thickness of the population and the susceptibility to infection; examples of development driven by movement, exchange, and relocation; speed and adequacy of public health surveillance and reaction measures).

Dense groupings of population, particularly in urban focuses harboring overcrowded informal settlements, can go about as foci for disease transmission and quicken the spread of pathogens. Also, social disparity, neediness, and natural relationship can build singular weakness to contamination fundamentally. Comorbidities, hunger, and caloric deficiencies debilitate a person's safe framework, while natural factors, for example, lack of clean water and sufficient sanitation, intensify transmission rates and increased morbidity and mortality. Every one of these components recommends that marginalized populations, including displaced people and individuals living in urban slums and casual settlements, likely face raised risks of morbidity and mortality during a pandemic.

A nation's reliance upon a capacity to shorten pandemic spread can be communicated utilizing a readiness file created by Oppenheim and others. The file shows worldwide variety in institutional availability to distinguish and react to an enormous scope outbreak of infectious illness. It draws on the IHR center limit measurements and other openly available cross-national pointers. In any case, it veers from the IHR measurements in its expansiveness and focuses on estimating basic and empowering institutional, infrastructural, and money related limits. For example, the following:

- Public wellbeing framework equipped for identifying, following, overseeing, and treating cases.

- Adequate physical and communications foundation to channel data and assets.
- Fundamental bureaucratic and public management capacities.
- Capacity to assemble financial assets to pay for infection reaction and accommodate the financial shock of the outbreak.
- Ability to embrace effective risk communications.

Well-prepared countries have compelling open organizations, strong economies, and satisfactory interest in the health sector. They have manufactured explicit capabilities basic to identifying and managing disease outbreaks, including surveillance, mass vaccination, and risk communications. Ineffectively arranged countries may experience the ill effects of political precariousness, powerless open organization, lacking assets for public health, and holes in crucial outbreak identification and response systems.

Burden of Pandemics

Evaluating the morbidity and mortality burden from pandemics represents a significant challenge. Although evaluations are available from authentic occasions, the correct record is inadequate and incomplete. To beat these holes in evaluating the recurrence and severity of pandemics, probabilistic demonstrating methods can expand the chronicled record with a large catalog of hypothetical, deductively conceivable, recreated pandemics that speak to a wide scope of potential situations. Modeling can also better record for changes that have happened since authentic occasions, for example, clinical advances, evolving socioeconomics, and moving travel designs.

Situation modeling of epidemics and pandemics can be accomplished through enormous scope PC simulations of worldwide spread, elements, and disease results of infection. These models consider the detail of parameters that may drive the probability of a spark (for instance, area and frequency) and determinants of severity (for instance, transmissibility and virulence). The models at that point recreate at an everyday time step the spread of disease from person to person via disease transmission elements and here and there using joining of long-range and short-go population developments. The models additionally can join moderation measures, regularity, stochastic procedures, and different elements that can shift during a pandemic. A huge number of these reenactments can be run with a wide variety of underlying conditions and ultimate results.

These huge numbers of simulations can be utilized to evaluate the weight of pandemics through a class of probabilistic demonstrating called catastrophe modeling, which the protection business uses to understand risks presented by inconsistent cataclysmic events like storms and earthquakes. At the point, when applied to pandemics, this methodology requires factually fitting appropriations of the parameters. These parameter circulations give weightings of the probability of various occasions. Through connected factual examination dependent on the parameter loads, situations are chosen for consideration in an occasion list of simulated pandemic events. A schematic diagram shows how the catastrophe modeling process is utilized to build up the event catalog.

Consequences of Pandemics

Health Impacts

The direct health impacts of pandemics can be harmful. During the Black Death, an expected 30–50 percent of the European population perished. All the more, as of late, the HIV/AIDS pandemic has killed more than 35 million people since 1981 (WHO Global Health Observatory information, http://www.who.int/gho/hiv/en).

Pandemics can excessively influence more youthful and even more economically active segments of the population. During flu pandemics (rather than seasonal outbreaks of flu), the horribleness and mortality age appropriations move to more youthful populations because more youthful individuals have lower insusceptibility than more established individuals, which altogether builds the long stretches of life lost. Besides, numerous infectious diseases can have chronic impacts, which can turn out to be progressively normal or far-reaching on account of a pandemic. For instance, Zika-related microcephaly has lifelong impacts on health and well-being.

The indirect health effects of pandemics can expand morbidity and mortality further. Drivers of indirect health impacts incorporate preoccupation or depletion of assets to give routine consideration and decreased access to routine consideration coming about because of an inability to travel, fear, or different variables.

Also, fear can lead to an upsurge of the "worried well" looking for extra consideration, and further troubling the human care system.

During the 2014 West Africa Ebola scourge, lack of routine care for malaria, HIV/AIDS, and tuberculosis prompted an expected 10,600 extra deaths in Guinea, Liberia, and Sierra Leone. This roundabout loss of life almost approached the 11,300 deaths directly brought about by Ebola in those countries. Also, redirection of assets, clinical assets, and staff prompted a 30 percent decline in routine youth vaccination rates in influenced countries. During the 2009 flu pandemic, a more prominent flood in emergency clinic affirmations for flu and pneumonia was related to measurably huge increments in deaths attributable from acute myocardial infarction and stroke. But, during a pandemic, recognizing which deaths are attributable to the pandemic itself and which are simply coincidental might be impossible.

During the 2014 West Africa Ebola pestilence, office closures because of understaffing and fear of getting the infection assumed an enormous job in lack of access to or evasion of routine medicinal services. One investigation of 45 public offices in Guinea found that the Ebola episode prompted a 31 percent decline in outpatient visits for routine maternal and child health services. Among kids under age five years, medical clinics saw a 60 percent decline in visits for loose bowels and a 58 percent decline in visits for acute respiratory illness (ARI). In contrast, health centers saw a 25 percent decline in visits for the runs and a 23 percent decline in visits for ARI. In Sierra Leone, visits to open offices for conceptive medicinal services fell by as much as 40 percent during the outbreak.

The availability of health care workers also reduced during a pandemic as a result of ailment, deaths, and fear driven non-attendance. Viral hemorrhagic fevers, for example, Ebola take a particularly serious cost for human services laborers, who face significant exposure to infectious material:

- During the main Ebola flare-up in the Democratic Republic of Congo in 1976 (at that point called Zaire), the Yambuku Mission Hospital was finished at the focal point of the outbreak because 11 off of the 17 staff members had died of the disease.
- During the Kikwit Ebola episode in 1995 in a similar nation, 24 percent of cases happened among known or possible health care workers.
- During the 2014 West Africa Ebola plague, medicinal services laborers experienced high death rates: 8 percent of doctors, nurses, and midwives

succumbed to Ebola in Liberia, 7 percent in Sierra Leone, and 1 percent in Guinea.

Regardless of whether health care workers don't bite the dust, their capacity to give care might be reduced. At the pinnacle of an extreme flu pandemic, up to 40 percent of medicinal services workers may be not able to report for obligation since they are sick themselves and need to think about sick relatives, as well as need to think about kids as a result of school closures; or they are afraid.

Economic Impacts

Pandemics can cause acute, short-term fiscal shocks just as longer-term damage to economic growth. Early-stage public health efforts to contain or limit outbreaks (for example, following contacts, executing isolates, and detaching infectious cases) involve critical human asset and staffing costs. As an outbreak grows, new offices may be built to deal with additional infectious cases; this, alongside expanding interest for consumables (clinical supplies, individual defensive hardware, and medications), can significantly build health system expenditures.

Reduced tax revenues may worsen fiscal stresses brought about by expanded uses, particularly in LMICs, where charge frameworks are more vulnerable, and government fiscal limitations are more extreme. This dynamic was obvious during the 2014 West Africa Ebola scourge in Liberia: while reaction costs flooded, financial movement eased back, and isolates and curfews decreased government ability to gather revenue.

During a mild or moderate pandemic, unaffected HICs can balance financial shocks by giving expanded official development assistance (ODA) to influenced nations, including direct budgetary support. However, during a serious pandemic where HICs stand up to the same financial stresses and might not be able or reluctant to give help, LMICs could confront bigger spending deficiencies, conceivably prompting debilitated general wellbeing reaction or cuts in another government spending.

The direct fiscal impacts of pandemics, for the most part, are little but comparative with the circuitous harm to financial movement and development. Negative financial development shocks are driven directly by work power decreases, which is brought about by disorder and mortality, and indirectly by fear instigated social changes. Fear shows itself through various social changes. As an investigation of the monetary effects of 2014, West Africa Ebola epidemic noted, "Fear of relationship with others reduces work power interest, closes work environments, disturbs transportation, propels a few governments to close land fringes, and limit the passage of residents from affected countries while motivating private leaders to upset exchange, travel, and trade by dropping planned business flights and decreasing delivery and cargo services." These impacts lessen work power investment well beyond the pandemic's direct morbidity and mortality impacts and constrict local and regional trade.

The indirect economic effect of pandemics has been evaluated essentially through calculable general balance simulations; the exact writing is less evolved. World Bank monetary recreations demonstrate that extreme pandemic could reduce world gross domestic product (GDP) by about 5 percent. The decrease, popular brought about by aversive behavior (for example, the evasion of movement, cafés, and open spaces, just as prophylactic working environment non-attendance), surpasses the financial effect of direct morbidity and mortality-associated absenteeism.

Social and Political Impacts

Proof recommends that pestilences and pandemics can have significant social and political outcomes, making conflicts among states and residents, dissolving state limit, driving population displacement, and increasing social pressure and discrimination.

Extreme pre-modern pandemics have been related to huge social and political change, driven by enormous mortality stuns and the resulting demographic shifts. Most eminently, deaths emerging from the presentation of smallpox and different infections to the Americas drove legitimately to the breakdown of numerous indigenous social orders and debilitated the indigenous people groups' establishments, as well as the military ability to the degree that they got powerless against European conquest. Consequent pandemics have not had such sensational consequences for political and social steadiness, principally because improvements in prevention and care have weakened the potential mortality stun.

Evidence suggests that scourges and pandemics can enhance existing political strains and spark distress, especially in delicate states with legacies of violence and weak institutions. During the 2014 West Africa Ebola plague, steps were taken to mitigate disease transmission; for example, the inconvenience of isolates and curfews by security powers was seen with doubt by the general population's fragments and restriction political leaders. This led directly to riots and rough conflicts with security powers. Inert political pressures from beforehand warring groups in Liberia also reemerged early in the pandemic. They were connected with risks to medicinal services workers just as attacks on public health personnel and facilities.

The Ebola epidemic also incredibly intensified political pressures in Guinea, Liberia, and Sierra Leone, with occupant government officials being blamed for utilizing the emergency and sickness control measures to cement political control and resistance figures blamed for hampering disease response efforts. While developing pressures didn't lead to a huge scope of political violence or insecurity, they complicate public health response efforts. In Sierra Leone, isolate in restriction overwhelmed areas was deferred, given worries that it would be viewed as politically motivated. In nations with elevated levels of political polarization, recent civil war, or weak establishments, sustained outbreaks could lead to more supported and testing political strains.

Patterns Affecting Pandemic Risk

In recent decades, a few patterns have influenced pandemic likelihood, readiness, and mitigation capacity. Different variables like population development, expanding urbanization, more significant interest for animal protein, greater travel, and availability between populace focus, living space loss, environmental change, and expanded collaborations at the human-creature interface influence the probability of pandemic occasions by expanding either the likelihood of a spark occasion or the potential spread of a pathogen. With the global population evaluated to arrive at 9.7 billion by 2050 and with movement and exchange consistently heightening, public health systems will have less time to recognize and contain a pandemic before it spreads.

Concerning poverty, the patterns are mixed. On the positive side, enormous gains in poverty reduction have decreased the number of people living in extreme poverty. This may weaken the mortality shock of a mild pandemic to some degree. On the negative side, extreme poverty is now concentrated in a few low-development, high-poverty countries. In such nations, progress in building health system capacity also has been far slower.

Moreover, for a subset of countries with endemically weak institutions, building institutional limits concerning complex tasks like pandemic relief and the reaction is probably going to be a moderate procedure much under the most idealistic assumptions. Huge numbers of these countries are in areas with high flash hazard, especially in Central and West Africa, and in this manner may stay powerless and require significant global help during a pandemic.

CONCLUSION

Planning for a pandemic is testing a result of a huge number of variables, huge numbers of which are extraordinary among natural events. Pandemics are rare occasions, and the risk of an event is impacted by anthropogenic changes in the natural environment. Furthermore, responsibility for preparedness is diffuse, and a considerable lot of the nations at the most serious risk has the most restricted ability to manage and mitigate pandemic risk. Unlike most other catastrophic events, pandemics don't remain geologically contained, and devastation can be relieved fundamentally through brief mediation. Thus, there are strong ethical and global health goals for building the ability to identify and react to pandemic threats, especially in countries with weak preparedness and high spark and spread risk. Expanding the trained health workforce also will build the ability to distinguish whether a specific population (for instance, human, livestock, or untamed life) is experiencing a pathogen with high pandemic risk. Expanding the health workforce also will improve the general flexibility of the well-being framework. This improvement can be applied to any crisis that outcomes in morbidity and mortality shocks.

Furthermore, building situational awareness will require a supported interest in infectious disease surveillance, crisis management, and risk communications systems. Interests in these limits are probably going to increase after pandemic or epidemic events and then decrease as different needs arise. Consequently, stable speculation to manufacture sustained capacity is critical. Throughout history, pandemics of infections, for example, cholera, plague, and flu, have assumed a significant job in molding human civic establishments. Instances of significant recorded pandemics incorporate the plague pandemic of the Byzantine Empire in the sixth century CE; the Black Death, which started in China and spread across Europe in the fourteenth century; and the flu pandemic of 1918–19, which began in the U.S. province of Kansas and spread to Europe, Asia, and islands in the South Pacific. Although pandemics are typically characterized by their event over a limited capacity to focus time, today, a few infectious diseases that continue at an elevated level of frequency happen on a worldwide scale and can be transmitted between people either straightforwardly or in a roundabout way. Such illnesses referred to in current pandemics incorporate AIDS, brought about by HIV (human immunodeficiency infection), which is transmitted directly between humans; and malaria brought about by parasites in the family Plasmodium, which are transmitted starting with one human, then onto the next by mosquitoes that feed on the blood of infected people.

www.ingramcontent.com/pod-product-compliance
Lightning Source LLC
Chambersburg PA
CBHW070905080526
44589CB00013B/1187